Oral and Maxillofacial Infections: 15 Unanswered Questions

Guest Editor

THOMAS R. FLYNN, DMD

ORAL AND MAXILLOFACIAL SURGERY CLINICS OF NORTH AMERICA

www.oralmaxsurgery.theclinics.com

Consulting Editor
RICHARD H. HAUG, DDS

November 2011 • Volume 23 • Number 4

SAUNDERS an imprint of ELSEVIER, Inc.

W.B. SAUNDERS COMPANY
A Division of Elsevier Inc.

1600 John F. Kennedy Blvd. • Suite 1800 • Philadelphia, PA 19103-2899

www.oralmaxsurgery.theclinics.com

ORAL AND MAXILLOFACIAL SURGERY CLINICS OF NORTH AMERICA Volume 23, Number 4
November 2011 ISSN 1042-3699, ISBN-13: 978-1-4557-7987-1

Editor: John Vassallo; j.vassallo@elsevier.com
Developmental Editor: Teia Stone

Oral and Maxillofacial Surgery Clinics of North America (ISSN 1042-3699) is published quarterly by Elsevier Inc., 360 Park Avenue South, New York, NY 10010-1710. Months of issue are February, May, August, and November. Business and Editorial Offices: 1600 John F. Kennedy Blvd., Suite 1800, Philadelphia, PA 19103-2899. Periodicals postage paid at New York, NY and additional mailing offices. Subscription prices are $329.00 per year for US individuals, $490.00 per year for US institutions, $147.00 per year for US students and residents, $383.00 per year for Canadian individuals, $583.00 per year for Canadian institutions, $441.00 per year for international individuals, $583.00 per year for international institutions and $200.00 per year for Canadian and foreign students/residents. To receive student/resident rate, orders must be accompanied by name or affiliated institution, date of term, and the *signature* of program/residency coordinator on institution letterhead. Orders will be billed at individual rate until proof of status is received. Foreign air speed delivery is included in all *Clinics* subscription prices. All prices are subject to change without notice. **POSTMASTER:** Send address changes to *Oral and Maxillofacial Surgery Clinics of North America,* Elsevier Periodicals Customer Service, 11830 Westline Industrial Drive, St. Louis, MO 63146. Tel: 1-800-654-2452 (U.S. and Canada); 314-447-8871 (outside U.S. and Canada). Fax: 314-447-8029. E-mail: journalscustomerservice-usa@elsevier.com (for print support); journalsonlinesupport-usa@elsevier.com (for online support).

Reprints. For copies of 100 or more, of articles in this publication, please contact the Commercial Reprints Department, Elsevier Inc., 360 Park Avenue South, New York, NY 10010-1710. Tel.: 212-633-3812; Fax: 212-462-1935; Email: reprints@elsevier.com.

Oral and Maxillofacial Surgery Clinics of North America is covered in MEDLINE/PubMed (*Index Medicus*).

Printed and bound by CPI Group (UK) Ltd, Croydon, CR0 4YY

Transferred to Digital Print 2011

Contributors

CONSULTING EDITOR

RICHARD H. HAUG, DDS
Carolinas Center for Oral Health,
Charlotte, North Carolina

GUEST EDITOR

THOMAS R. FLYNN, DMD
Formerly, Associate Professor of Oral and
Maxillofacial Surgery, Department of Oral and
Maxillofacial Surgery, Harvard School of Dental
Medicine, Boston, Massachusetts; Currently,
Private Practice, Reno, Nevada

AUTHORS

SHAHID R. AZIZ, DMD, MD, FACS
Associate Professor, Department of Oral and
Maxillofacial Surgery, University of Medicine
and Dentistry of New Jersey, Newark,
New Jersey

JOEL K. CURÉ, MD
Professor of Radiology, Department
of Radiology, University of Alabama
at Birmingham, Birmingham, Alabama

JOSEPH R. DEATHERAGE, DMD, MD, FACD
Private Practice, Face and Jaw Surgery Center,
Bismarck, North Dakota

THOMAS B. DODSON, DMD, MPH
Professor of Oral and Maxillofacial Surgery,
Visiting (Attending) Surgeon and Director,
Department of Oral and Maxillofacial Surgery,
Center for Applied Clinical Investigation,
Massachusetts General Hospital and Harvard
School of Dental Medicine, Boston,
Massachusetts

THOMAS R. FLYNN, DMD
Formerly, Associate Professor of Oral and
Maxillofacial Surgery, Department of Oral and
Maxillofacial Surgery, Harvard School of Dental
Medicine, Boston, Massachusetts; Currently,
Private Practice, Reno, Nevada

DREW B. HAVARD, DMD
Resident, Department of Oral and Maxillofacial
Surgery, Baylor College of Dentistry, Texas
A&M Health Science Center, Dallas, Texas

STEVEN M. HOLMES, DDS
Risk Management Consultant, OMS National
Insurance Company, Rosemont, Illinois

STEVEN R. IZZO, DDS
Associate Director, Department of Dental/Oral
and Maxillofacial Surgery, Kings County
Hospital Center, Brooklyn, New York

ANKUR JOHRI, DDS, MD
Senior Resident, Division of Oral and
Maxillofacial Surgery, University of
Connecticut Health Center, Farmington,
Connecticut

**GERARD F. KOORBUSCH, DDS, MBA,
FACD, FICD**
Private Practice, Face and Jaw Surgery Center,
Bismarck, North Dakota

DANIEL M. LASKIN, DDS, MS
Professor and Chairman Emeritus, Department
of Oral and Maxillofacial Surgery, Virginia
Commonwealth University School of Dentistry
and VCU Medical Center, Richmond, Virginia

STEWART K. LAZOW, MD, DDS, FACS
Professor, Vice Chairman, and Residency Program Director, Department of Dental/Oral and Maxillofacial Surgery, Kings County Hospital Center–State University of New York, Brooklyn, New York

FRANCISCO M. MARTY, MD
Assistant Professor of Medicine, Division of Infectious Diseases, Brigham and Women's Hospital, Dana-Farber Cancer Institute, Harvard Medical School, Boston, Massachusetts

RICHARD NIEDERMAN, DMD, MA
Director, Center for Evidence-Based Dentistry, The Forsyth Institute, Cambridge, Massachusetts

STEFAN PALMASON, DMD
Oral Medicine Resident, Division of Oral Medicine and Dentistry, Brigham and Women's Hospital; Department of Oral Medicine, Infection and Immunity, Harvard School of Dental Medicine, Boston, Massachusetts

JOSEPH F. PIECUCH, DMD, MD
Clinical Professor, Division of Oral and Maxillofacial Surgery, University of Connecticut Health Center, Farmington, Connecticut

J. MICHAEL RAY, DDS
Assistant Professor, Department of Oral and Maxillofacial Surgery, Baylor College of Dentistry, Texas A&M Health Science Center, Dallas, Texas

DEREK RICHARDS, BDS, MSc, DPPH, FDS (DPH)
Director, Centre for Evidence-Based Dentistry, University of Oxford, Oxford, United Kingdom

RABIE M. SHANTI, DMD, MD
Resident, Department of Oral and Maxillofacial Surgery, University of Medicine and Dentistry of New Jersey, Newark, New Jersey

BASEL SHARAF, DDS, MD
Assistant Clinical Professor, Department of Surgery, School of Medicine and Biomedical Sciences, University at Buffalo, State University of New York, Buffalo, New York

SRINIVAS M. SUSARLA, DMD, MD, MPH
Resident, Department of Oral and Maxillofacial Surgery, Massachusetts General Hospital, Boston, Massachusetts

NATHANIEL S. TREISTER, DMD, DMSc
Associate Surgeon, Division of Oral Medicine and Dentistry, Brigham and Women's Hospital; Assistant Professor of Oral Medicine, Department of Oral Medicine, Infection and Immunity, Harvard School of Dental Medicine, Boston, Massachusetts

R. GILBERT TRIPLETT, DDS, PhD
Regents Professor, Department of Oral and Maxillofacial Surgery, Baylor College of Dentistry, Texas A&M Health Science Center, Dallas, Texas

DEBRA K. UDEY, BA
Vice President, Risk Management, OMS National Insurance Company, Rosemont, Illinois

DAVID VAZQUEZ, DMD
Chief Resident, Department of Dental/Oral and Maxillofacial Surgery, Kings County Hospital Center, Brooklyn, New York

Contents

From Celsus' first reports of rubor, calor, dolor, tumor, and functio laesa, has come an understanding of inflammation's manifestations at the organ, tissue, vascular, cellular, genetic, and molecular levels. Molecular medicine now raises the opposite question: can local oral infections and their inflammatory mediators increase systemic morbidity or mortality? From these perspectives we examine the clinical evidence relating caries, periodontal disease, and pericoronitis to systemic disease. Widespread affirmation of an oral-systemic linkage remains elusive, raising sobering cautions.

Most infections of the head and neck and virtually all of those encountered in the practice of dentistry are caused by bacteria that are organized into biofilms. A biofilm is a complex, usually multispecies, highly communicative community of bacteria that is surrounded by a polymeric matrix. Treatment of these types of infections with traditional antibiotics alone is ineffective, and surgical removal of diseased tissue is still necessary.

Immediate extraction of teeth in the setting of an acute infection has shown to be beneficial for many reasons. It results in faster resolution of the infection, decreased pain, and earlier return of function and oral intake. The risk of seeding the infection into deeper spaces by performing immediate extraction is low.

Deep neck infections are infections (either abscess or cellulitis) that are within the potential spaces and fascial planes of the head and neck. Deep neck infections should not be ignored, and no surgeon should underestimate the necessity of appropriate and timely treatment of deep neck infections due to the serious and potentially life-threatening nature of these infections. This article discusses and reviews the literature with regard to a question that has long been debated in the surgical literature, "Should we wait for the development of an abscess before performing incision and drainage?"

In the everyday practice of oral and maxillofacial surgeons, empiric antibiotics are prescribed in the face of uncertainty. Is there a highly resistant organism present? Are the old-line antibiotics no longer effective? Should a broad-spectrum antibiotic be used just to cover all the bases in this case? The surprising result of this systematic review is that when combined with appropriate surgery, the usual antibiotics are all effective. Safety and cost become the differentiating factors in this clinical decision.

Generally, antibiotics should not be required before the removal of erupted carious or periodontally involved teeth unless a significant risk of postoperative infection is present. The decision to use prophylactic antibiotics in noninfected cases should also be based on whether patients have any significant medical risk factors that could adversely affect their humoral and cellular defense mechanisms, and whether any systemic risks are associated with the bacteremia that accompanies tooth extraction. This article discusses the various indications for using prophylactic antibiotics in patients having erupted teeth extracted based on a consideration of these factors.

Surgical removal of impacted third molars remains the most common procedure performed by oral and maxillofacial surgeons. Given the abundance of host bacteria within the operative sites, surgical site infections are among the most common complications of third molar removal, with an estimated frequency of 1% to 30%. In this setting, significant controversy has surrounded the use of prophylactic antibiotics in the surgical management of impacted third molars. This article provides a comprehensive review of the available data on antibiotic prophylaxis in impacted third molar surgery and offers specific recommendations on antibiotic use.

The use of prophylactic antibiotics in implant dentistry is controversial. Given the known risks of antibiotic treatment and lack of consensus on using antibiotics at the time of implant insertion, the purpose of this article was to review available studies on use of perioperative prophylactic antibiotics at the time of implant placement and to provide evidence-based recommendations for antibiotic use. The reviewed studies suggest that a single preoperative dose of 2 g amoxicillin 1 hour before implant placement or 1 g amoxicillin 1 hour preoperatively and 500 mg 4 times daily 2 days postoperatively can reduce the rate of implant failure.

More than 30 million pounds of antibiotics are used in the United States per year, more than 90% for nontherapeutic purposes in animals. Environmental contamination by trace amounts of antibiotics and highly resistant bacteria can lead to resistant infections in humans. Oral and maxillofacial infections are largely mediated by biofilms, which are resistant to antibiotics. Primary treatment is surgical debridement, removal of the cause of the infection, and drainage of pus. Current best practices indicate the use of antibiotics as adjunctive therapy to surgery only when regional, distant, or systemic spread of the infection is a significant risk.

Oral and Maxillofacial Surgery Clinics of North America

FORTHCOMING ISSUES

February 2012

Rhinoplasty: Current Therapy
Shahrokh C. Bagheri, DMD, MD, FACS,
Husain Ali Khan, DMD, MD and
Angelo Cuzalina, MD, *Guest Editors*

May 2012

**Surgery of the Nose and Paranasal Sinuses:
Principles and Concepts**
Orrett Ogle, DDS and Harry Dym, DDS,
Guest Editors

August 2012

Pediatric Maxillofacial Surgery
Bruce B. Horswell, MD, DDS and
Michael S. Jaskolka, MD, DDS,
Guest Editors

RECENT ISSUES

August 2011

Complications in Dentoalveolar Surgery
Dennis-Duke R. Yamashita, DDS and
James P. McAndrews, DDS,
Guest Editors

May 2011

Dental Implants
Ole T. Jensen, DDS, MS,
Guest Editor

February 2011

Reoperative Oral and Maxillofacial Surgery
Luis G. Vega, DDS and
Rui Fernandes, DMD, MD,
Guest Editors

RELATED INTEREST

Infectious Disease Clinics of North America, December 2009 (Vol. 23, No. 4)
Antibacterial Therapy and Newer Agents
Keith S. Kaye, MD, MPH and Donald Kaye, MD, *Guest Editors*

THE CLINICS ARE NOW AVAILABLE ONLINE!
Access your subscription at:
www.theclinics.com

Preface

Oral and Maxillofacial Infections: 15 Unanswered Questions

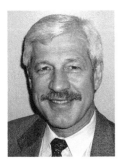

Thomas R. Flynn, DMD
Guest Editor

In all affairs it's a healthy thing now and then to hang a question mark on the things you have long taken for granted.
— *Bertrand Russell (1872–1970)*

Every day as clinicians, we must make decisions in the face of uncertainty. We have so many questions, and so few answers. Are there antibiotic-resistant organisms in this infection? Should I do surgery now, later, or not at all? Does this patient really need a prophylactic antibiotic? Is this really an osteomyelitis? Might this infection spread into the brain or migrate into the heart? Which antibiotic is best for this patient?

Nonetheless, we must act in the present in order to protect our patient's future. Therefore, we make rules. We accept the rules we were taught without question. They give us certainty in the face of no information.

This issue of the *Oral and Maxillofacial Surgery Clinics of North America* examines 15 questions that linger in the back of our heads as we make our daily decisions. Some of those questions have already been answered with good research, yet the knowledge is not widely appreciated. Some of these questions have not been answered by definitive research. Yet they have been explored, and we do have limited answers for them.

We have attempted, to the best of our ability, to "hang a question mark on the things you have long taken for granted," as Bertrand Russell said, and to examine the best available scientific evidence on the unanswered questions about the infections we treat every day.

You will see references throughout this issue to "levels of evidence." Where possible, we have tried to rate the available evidence on this scale. In simplified fashion, the dependability of the scientific

Evidence Level	Type of Research
1a	Meta-analyses and systematic reviews of multiple randomized clinical trials (RCT)
1b	Individual RCTs
2	Quasi-experimental research: cohort studies, low-quality RCTs, outcomes research
3	Case-control studies
4	Case series
5	Expert opinion, practice guidelines, experimental laboratory research

Oral Maxillofacial Surg Clin N Am 23 (2011) ix–x
doi:10.1016/j.coms.2011.08.002
1042-3699/11/$ – see front matter

oralmaxsurgery.theclinics.com

evidence of causation can be graded according to the following table adapted from multiple sources. The first article in this issue fully explains evidence-based dentistry and evaluates the evidence on whether oral inflammation plays a significant role in systemic disease.

This is also very much a generational issue of the *Oral and Maxillofacial Surgery Clinics of North America*. The authors of these articles range from its pioneers, to its giants, to its young lions, and to its rising stars. If you do not know the names of these contributors, learn them. You will see them again; so much of the future of our specialty is in their hands. By asking and answering these questions to the best of our current knowledge, they have done us all a great service. They have put into action the principle so beautifully stated below by Sophocles so long ago.

Knowledge must come through action; you can have no test which is not fanciful, save by trial.
—Sophocles, 496 BC-406 BC

The contributors to this issue have done us a great service. Thank you, colleagues!

Thomas R. Flynn, DMD
1055 Waverly Drive
Reno, NV 89519, USA

E-mail address:
thomasrflynndmd@gmail.com

What is Evidence-Based Dentistry, and Do Oral Infections Increase Systemic Morbidity or Mortality?

Richard Niederman, DMD, MA[a],*,
Derek Richards, BDS, MSc, DPPH, FDS (DPH)[b]

KEYWORDS

- Evidence-based dentistry • Oral infections
- Molecular medicine • Inflammation

The goal of evidence-based health care, and more specifically evidence-based dentistry (EBD), is to improve health. The mechanism for accomplishing this is by integrating: the current best evidence with clinical judgment, and the patient needs, values, and circumstances.[1]

Over the last 20 years, clinicians at the Institute of Healthcare Improvement (IHI) successfully developed, tested, and implemented a process to continually improve health. The concepts IHI employs derive from the quality improvement methods embedded in Toyota's Lean Processing (waste reduction), and Motorola's 6-Sigma (variation reduction) programs. And, interestingly, Toyota and Motorola developed their systems from the work of Walter Shewhart and Edwards Deming, who first applied quality improvement methods at Bell Telephone to improve the reliability of their transmission systems.

Quality improvement programs ask 3 conceptual questions:

1. What do I want to improve?
2. What can I do to improve?
3. How will I know that I improved?

In healthcare, the first and third questions require assessments of patient values and clinical judgment, respectively, and can be characterized as "know what" and "know how."[2]

The second question is the challenge addressed here. To improve health, one needs access to the current best evidence. Yet, it is highly unlikely that practicing clinicians can stay current. Estimates from 10 years ago indicated that more than 800 clinical articles are published annually in oral and maxillofacial surgery, and that the number of articles was increasing at approximately 10% per year. In other words, to stay current, a clinician would need to identify, obtain, read, appraise, and decide whether to implement more than 2 articles per day, 365 days per year for the rest of their clinical lives.[3] This was a Herculean task 10 years ago, more so today, and one unlikely to be fulfilled by most clinicians. Making clinical life more complicated is deciding among conflicting results of clinical publications, which lead to variability in clinical care (see below).

Fortunately, knowledge creators provide guidance for this in the context of an evidence pyramid and tools to use it (**Fig. 1**). In this pyramid, the higher the level of evidence, the more likely the evidence is to predict cause–effect and what would occur in one's practice. And conversely, the lower the level of evidence, the

a Center for Evidence-Based Dentistry, The Forsyth Institute, 245 First Street, Cambridge, MA 02142, USA
b Centre for Evidence-based Dentistry, University of Oxford, Rewley House, 1 Wellington Square, Oxford OX1 2JA, UK
* Corresponding author.
E-mail address: rniederman1@gmail.com

Oral Maxillofacial Surg Clin N Am 23 (2011) 491–496
doi:10.1016/j.coms.2011.07.001
1042-3699/11/$ – see front matter © 2011 Elsevier Inc. All rights reserved.

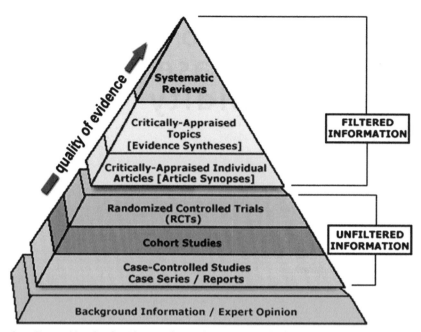

Fig. 1. Types of studies and levels of evidence. The evidence pyramid is broken into 3 parts. Filtered information is the highest level. It is so-called secondary research. These reports systematically search for, critically appraise, distill, and present the results of primary research—unfiltered information. The highest evidence level, with the highest likelihood of predicting what would occur in one's own practice, and the least probability of bias, is the systematic review. Conversely, the lowest level of evidence, with the least likelihood of predicting what would occur in one's practice, and the highest probability of bias is background information (eg, laboratory and animal studies, cross-sectional epidemiologic studies, and expert opinion or narrative reviews). (© Copyright 2006 Trustees of Dartmouth College and Yale University. All rights reserved. Produced by Jan Glover, Dave Izzo, Karen Odato, and Lei Wang; used with permission.)

less likely it is to predict cause–effect and what would occur in one's practice. In other words, a higher level of evidence trumps a lower level of evidence. The figure captures both the concept of a fair test of treatments and distills the historical evolution of this concept from 1550 BCE, through Sir Francis Bacon's scientific method to the current time.[4]

The highest level of evidence is a systematic review of clinical trials. Conversely, the lowest level of evidence is the traditional narrative review or expert opinion. Between the 2 types of reviews are unfiltered primary reports of clinical trials and filtered secondary reports that distill information from the primary reports.

Note that cross-sectional epidemiology, laboratory, and animal studies are not considered. Cross-sectional epidemiologic studies, because they occur at 1 point in time, cannot predict cause–effect relationships. However, they can be and are used to identify associations. Specifically, it is these cross-sectional studies that have been used to propose an association between oral infections, inflammation, and systemic disease.

VARIATION IN CARE AND CONFLICTING TRIAL OUTCOMES

The nonpartisan Congressional Budget Office identifies variation in care and rising health care costs as "the central fiscal challenge facing the country."[5] Variation in healthcare is chronicled yearly in the Dartmouth Atlas of Healthcare (www.dartmouthatlas.org/default.php). Its findings indicate that extraordinary variations in care and outcomes occur across the United States. Consequently, the Congressional Budget Office recommends that improved quality of care can be achieved by reducing the overuse of inappropriate or ineffective interventions, increasing the underuse of effective interventions, and eliminating misuse or medical errors.

One example of this variation and the value of the evidence pyramid comes from the work of Ioannidis, who quantitatively examined the occurrence of conflicting trial results. He found that most published clinical research findings are false.[6] He then examined the cause and found the trials using methods that were more prone to bias were largely contradicted by trials using methods that were less prone to bias.[7] In other words, epidemiologic studies were largely contradicted by subsequent case–control studies, and these were largely contradicted by cohort study designs. Finally, trials using randomization and masking were largely unchallenged.[7] Unfortunately, however, persistent clinical use of contraindicated concepts and interventions continues long after more definitive studies are published.[8] This leads to significant variation in care.

EVIDENCE AND STANDARDS OF CARE

The US Supreme Court recognizes the utility of the evidence pyramid and its probability to predict causality.[9] Currently, the World Health Organization, the US Department of Health and Human Services, and its subsidiary organizations (eg, Centers for Disease Control and Prevention [CDC], the National Institutes of Health) all support evidence-based healthcare. Similarly, independent professional organizations including the US Institute of Medicine, the American Medical Association, the American Dental Association (ADA), and the Federation Dentaire Internationale all support evidence-based healthcare. Because of this issue, in 2010 the ADA's Council on Dental Accreditation mandated that all US oral health training programs include EBD training.

At the same time, the definition of standard of care is evolving. It is evolving from the practice patterns of local communities and specialized clinicians toward alignment with international standards for health care evidence. The evolving definition of standards of care brings with it concomitant changes in the definition of benefits and risk.

PERCEIVED DEFICITS OF EBD

Iconoclasts and traditionalists will dismiss EBD with one or both of two thoughts:

(1) It is too technically difficult to implement, and cannot be implemented perfectly (the converse is also true: perfection is the enemy of good).
(2) All the evidence is not in, and even if it were, it still would not be definitive (this has been true throughout history and will continue to be true).

Examples of implementation avoidance in the face of good clinical evidence abound. The two classic examples of underuse come from James Lind and Ignaz Semmelweis. James Lind, in 1747, carried out the first controlled trial and demonstrated that citrus prevents scurvy. It took 50 years for the British Navy to mandate the use

of citrus, and another 200 years for citrus to become the Navy's standard scurvy preventive measure (www.jameslindlibrary.org). In 1847, Semmelweis found that the incidence of puerperal fever could be dramatically reduced by hand washing.[10,11] Yet, more than 150 years later, the CDC and the Joint Commission found it necessary to publish hand hygiene guidelines, and methods for implementation and assessment.[10,11]

ORAL AND SYSTEMIC DISEASE

Caries, periodontal disease, and pericoronitis are oral infections that stimulate an inflammatory response. From the fact that these infections and their inflammatory mediators can systemically disseminate arose the current concepts of an oral–systemic disease relationship.

The oral–systemic disease relationship concept however, is over 100 years old. This concept was previously termed the focal theory of infection. The focal theory hypothesized that an infection and toxins in one part of the body can spread to distant organs and compromise them. The modern origins derive from the studies of Robert Koch (from whom are derived Koch's postulates) and his student Willoughby Miller, whose publication titled: The Human Mouth as a Focus of Infection (1891),[12] galvanized generations of dentists and physicians. In the United States the physician Frank Billings,[13] in his 1916 Lane Lectures at Stanford University titled Focal Infections, laid the ground work for extractions of teeth and removal of tonsils to treat systemic diseases. The introduction starts:

> *"The importance of the etiologic relation of focal infection to systemic diseases has been a subject of study in the clinical material…for the past twelve or more years…The conclusions based upon the research were not made until a critical survey of the work and the results were investigated by other qualified clinicians, pathologists, and research workers."*

The 1923 text book Dental Infections, Oral and Systemic by Weston Price,[14] who founded the research section of the American Dental Association, set the standard of care for tooth extractions as the treatment of choice for both oral and systemic maladies.

In 1938 and 1940, the tide changed with the publication of human clinical studies that tested these concepts, and found them to be unsubstantiated.[15,16] The ADA followed suit,[17] and for almost 40 years the focal infection theory lay fallow. Historically, clinical trials trumped observations.

This changed when 3 groups, using cross-sectional studies, case–control, or cohort methods, found that cardiovascular disease and preterm low birth weight were associated with periodontal disease.[18–21] More recently, the death of Diamante Driver from a disseminating oral infection was a widely reported verification of this concept. The inductive extrapolation from these and other studies is the following: if oral infections and their inflammatory mediators disseminate systemically, and cause morbidity and/or mortality, then one must provide treatment of oral infections to prevent systemic maladies.

This hypothesis is appealingly straight-forward. It makes biological, clinical, and intuitive sense, and there are cogent supporting examples. This interest accounts for typical press reports in January 2011:

> "Healthy Gums, Healthy Lungs: Maintaining Healthy Teeth and Gums May Reduce Risk for Pneumonia, Chronic Obstructive Pulmonary Disease" (http://www.sciencedaily.com/releases/2011/01/110118143224.htm)
>
> "Tooth Loss May Be Linked to Memory Loss. Gum infection may cause inflammation that affects the brain, researcher suggests." (http://www.nlm.nih.gov/medlineplus/news/fullstory_107298.html).

On examination, it turns out that both of the press-reported studies are cross-sectional, which can only generate associations. They do not demonstrate cause–effect. And as indicated in the evidence pyramid, they are at the bottom rung, background information.

To critically examine the current status of the cause–effect relationships between oral infections and systemic disease, the authors queried MEDLINE in January 2011 (**Table 1**). The search identified 3950 reviews, of which 103 were systematic reviews with meta-analysis. These reviews are based on 1167 randomized controlled trials and 1993 clinical trials. Examination of the systematic reviews with meta-analysis identified 6 trials addressing pregnancy, 7 addressing coronary heart disease/stroke, 8 addressing diabetes, and 1 addressing pneumonia/chronic obstructive pulmonary disease.

The summary statements for all of the reviews were similarly guarded. The most cautious, a systematic review appraising randomized controlled trials examining the effect of periodontal therapy on preterm low birth weight stated: "Results of this meta-analysis do not support the hypothesis that periodontal therapy reduces preterm birth and LBW [low birth weight] indices."[22] The least tentative, a systematic review appraising randomized controlled trials testing the effect of periodontal therapy on glycemic control stated: "There is some evidence of improvement in metabolic control in people with diabetes, after treating periodontal disease."[23] However, Simpson and colleagues go on to offer a very cautionary note: "There are few studies available, and individually these lacked the power to detect a significant effect."

Table 1
Search strategy and results

Search Step	Search Strategy	# Publications
1.	Cardiovascular diseases (congenital, hereditary, or neonatal diseases or abnormalities) or digestive system diseases or endocrine system diseases or eye diseases or female urogenital diseases or pregnancy complications (hemic or lymphatic and diseases) or immune system diseases or male urogenital diseases or musculoskeletal diseases or nervous system diseases (nutritional or metabolic diseases) or otorhinolaryngologic diseases (pathological and conditions, signs, or symptoms) or respiratory tract diseases (skin or connective tissue diseases)	7,900,989
2.	Caries or periodontal disease or pericoronitis	101,394
3.	#1 and #2	36,155
4.	#3 Limits: review	3950
5.	#3 Limits: meta-analysis	103
6.	#3 Limits: randomized controlled trial	1167
7.	#3 Limits: clinical trial	1,993

As straight-forward and clear as these summary statements are, and they represent the current highest level of evidence, they contradict the appealing intuitive hypothesis that oral disease has an adverse effect on systemic health. Thus clinicians will naturally balance the conclusions from a handful of systematic reviews against the 3950 narrative reviews on the same topics, and their own clinical experiences that identify an association between oral and systemic diseases. The sheer number of papers, the biological elegance of the arguments, and the potential impact, if correct, are powerfully alluring. Interestingly, however, the narrative reviews largely base their conclusions on studies of surrogate outcome measures (eg, bacteria and inflammatory mediators associated with oral infections and systemic disease), not on the primary outcome of actual disease. As pointed out by Ioannidis, in the evolution of the focal theory of infection, over-reliance on lower levels of evidence can lead to false conclusions.

Five other points are important to note. First, the periodontal interventions that have been tried so far are scaling and root planning to treat periodontal disease. Clinical investigators have not yet examined the potential benefits of antimicrobial agents that have been found to be very effective in treating periodontal infections (eg, amoxicillin + metronidazole[24]) and then determined the effects on systemic disease. Second, as pointed out by Carl Sagan, absence of evidence is not evidence of absence. Clinical scientists may have not yet generated the key clinical question or key clinical test. Third, reliance on lower levels of evidence can lead to false conclusions, and the persistence of these incorrect conclusions can continue long after definitive studies are published.[6–8] Fourth, today's litigious society, with legal practices focusing on malpractice, and the Office Management and Budget Report focusing on overuse, underuse, and misuse,[5] suggest a word of caution. That is, treatment of oral disease is clearly beneficial in and of itself. However, current evidence does not support oral treatment for the prevention of systemic morbidity or mortality. Fifth, given the dynamic state of discussion around asymptomatic third molar extraction guidelines,[25] the benefits,[26] the risks,[27] the controversies,[28] and the actuarial life tables,[29] one might want to consider decision cut points for prophylactic care.

REFERENCES

1. Straus SE, Haynes RB, Richardson WS, et al. Evidence-based medicine. 3rd edition. Philadelphia: Elsevier Health Sciences; 2005.
2. Niederman R, Leitch J. Know what and know how: knowledge creation in clinical practice. J Dent Res 2006;85:296–7.
3. Niederman R, Chen L, Murzyn L, et al. Benchmarking the dental randomized controlled literature on MEDLINE. Evid Based Dent 2002;3:5–9.
4. Available at: www.JamesLindLibrary.org. Accessed July 22, 2011.
5. Orszag P. The overuse, underuse, and misuse of health care. Washington, DC: Congressional Budget Office; 2008.
6. Ioannidis JP. Contradicted and initially stronger effects in highly cited clinical research. JAMA 2005;294(2):218–28.
7. Ioannidis JP. Why most published research findings are false. PLoS Med 2005;2(8):e124.
8. Tatsioni A, Bonitsis NG, Ioannidis JP. Persistence of contradicted claims in the literature. JAMA 2007; 298(21):2517–26.
9. Daubert v Merrell Dow Pharmaceuticals, Inc., 509 US 579, 589 (1993).
10. Boyce JM, Pittet D. Guideline for hand hygiene in healthcare settings. Recommendations of the Healthcare Infection Control Practices Advisory Committee and the HICPAC/SHEA/APIC/IDSA Hand Hygiene Task Force. MMWR Recomm Rep 2002;51(RR-16):1–45.
11. Measuring hand hygiene adherence: overcoming the challenges. Oakbrook (IL): Joint Commission; 2009.
12. Miller WD. The human mouth as a focus of infection. Dent Cosmos 1891;33:689, 789, 913.
13. Billings F. Focal infection. The lane medical lectures. New York: D. Appleton and Company; 1916.
14. Price WA. Dental infections, oral and systemic. Cleveland (OH): Penton; 1923.
15. Cecil DL, Angevine DM. Clinical and experimental observations of focal infection, with an analysis of 200 cases of rheumatoid arthritis. Ann Intern Med 1938;5:577–84.
16. Reimann HA, Havens WP. Focal infection and systemic disease: a critical appraisal. The case against indiscriminate removal of theeth and tonsils clinical leture at St. Louis Session. JAMA 1940;114:1–6.
17. Eastlick K. An evaluation of the effect of dental focal infection on health. J Am Dent Assoc 1951;42:609–97.
18. Beck J, Garcia R, Heiss G, et al. Periodontal disease and cardiovascular disease. J Periodontol 1996; 67(Suppl 10):1123–37.
19. DeStefano F, Anda RF, Kahn HS, et al. Dental disease and risk of coronary heart disease and mortality. BMJ 1993;306:688–91.
20. Mattila KJ, Nieminen MS, Valtonen VV, et al. Association between dental health and acute myocardial infarction. BMJ 1989;298(6676):779–81.
21. Offenbacher S, Katz V, Fertik G, et al. Periodontal infection as a possible risk factor for preterm low birth weight. J Periodontol 1996;67(Suppl 10): 1103–13.

22. Fogacci MF, Vettore M, Thomé Leão AT. The effect of periodontal therapy on preterm low birth weight: a meta-analysis. Obstet Gynecol 2011;117:153–65.

23. Simpson TC, Needleman I, Wild SH, et al. Treatment of periodontal disease for glycaemic control in people with diabetes. Cochrane Database Syst Rev 2010;5:CD004714.

24. van Winkelhoff AJ, Tijhof CJ, de Graaff J. Microbiological and clinical results of metronidazole plus amoxicillin therapy in *Actinobacillus actinomycetemcomitans*-associated periodontitis. J Periodontol 1992;63:52–7.

25. Guidance on the extraction of wisdom teeth. Technology Appraisal Guidance. London: National Institute of Clinical Excellence; 2000.

26. Rosemont. White paper on third molar data. American Association of Oral and Maxillofaical Surgeons; 2007. Available at: www.aaoms.org/docs/third_molar_white_paper.pdf. Accessed July 22, 2011.

27. Jerjes W, Upile T, Nhembe F, et al. Experience in third molar surgery: an update. Br Dent J 2010; 209(1):E1.

28. Friedman JW. The prophylactic extraction of third molars: a public health hazard. Am J Public Health 2007;97:1554–9.

29. Fernandes MJ, Ogden GR, Pitts NB, et al. Actuarial life-table analysis of lower impacted wisdom teeth in general dental practice. Community Dent Oral Epidemiol 2010;38(1):58–67.

What is the Role of Biofilms in Severe Head and Neck Infections?

J. Michael Ray, DDS*, R. Gilbert Triplett, DDS, PhD

KEYWORDS

- Biofilm • Odontogenic infection • Peri-implantitis
- Osteonecrosis • Osteomyelitis

Although microbial biofilms were described decades ago, only recently have their importance in nature and their role in human infectious diseases been appreciated. Biofilms are well known to cause the infections of cystic fibrosis, joint prostheses, endocarditis, and virtually all implanted devices.[1] It is estimated that 65% to 80% of all human bacterial infections are related to bacterial biofilms.[2] Biofilms are described as matrix-embedded microbial populations, adherent to each other and/or to surfaces or interfaces.[3] These surfaces can be naturally occurring, such as bone, endothelial linings, and teeth, or inert surfaces such as implanted devices. Most bacteria in nature do not occur as free-floating organisms, but rather are organized as a "structured community of bacterial cells enclosed in a self-produced polymeric matrix."[4] This ability to attach to a surface is an important bacterial survival mechanism that contributes to the difficulty in curing infections caused by biofilms.

A biofilm develops as planktonic, or "free-floating," bacteria come in contact and attach to a surface. Bacteria themselves account for only a fraction of the total biofilm volume, usually about 15%.[5] The remainder is mostly an extracellular matrix composed of an exopolysaccharide matrix produced by the resident bacteria. The bacteria begin to lay down the exopolysaccharide almost immediately after attachment. This exopolysaccharide matrix allows for a means of trapping necessary nutrients from its surroundings and provides some protection against chemical and biological threats. More importantly, it provides a mechanism for cohesion of microbial clumps and adhesion to surfaces. Within this extracellular polymeric matrix, interconnecting channels separate the microbial clusters and allow for water and nutrient flow, for waste removal, and for the potential spread of the bacteria within the biofilm (**Fig. 1**). Quorum sensing is a method of intercellular and interspecies communication used to make decisions regarding gene expression based on environmental influences,[6] which is accomplished using signaling molecules secreted by neighboring cells. Once a threshold of inducer signals has been reached, receptors on neighboring cells are activated and the desired gene is expressed by the biofilm community, for example, detachment of a clump of bacteria or activation of a resistance mechanism.[5]

Most biofilms are not populated by a single species of bacteria. Rather, most exist as a heterogeneous and highly organized "community" in which the resident bacterial species interact with each other.[5] Although conventional systemic and topical antibiotics may be effective at killing planktonic bacteria, bacterial species within biofilms possess a unique resistance to antimicrobials that is quite different from classic antimicrobial resistance. In addition to the physical barrier the exopolysaccharide may provide, these metabolic

The authors have nothing to disclose.
Department of Oral and Maxillofacial Surgery, Baylor College of Dentistry, Texas A&M Health Science Center, 3302 Gaston Avenue, Dallas, TX 75246, USA
* Corresponding author.
E-mail address: mray@bcd.tamhsc.edu

Oral Maxillofacial Surg Clin N Am 23 (2011) 497–505
doi:10.1016/j.coms.2011.07.002
1042-3699/11/$ – see front matter © 2011 Elsevier Inc. All rights reserved.

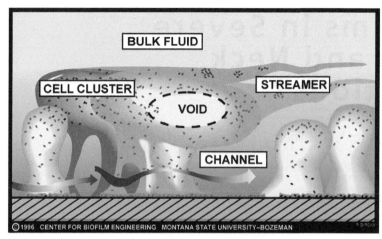

Fig. 1. Conceptual cartoon illustrating the heterogeneity of biofilm structure, showing bacterial clusters, voids, streamers, and water channels. (*Courtesy of* P. Dirckx; © MSU Center for Biofilm Engineering; with permission.)

and molecular interactions among different species in the community allow for the transfer of genetic and signaling information and differences in gene expression, which lead to this unique resistance of biofilm bacteria to eradication by conventional antibiotic therapy.[2] While surface bacteria may be killed, bacteria deep within the biofilm remain unaffected. Many of the deeper bacteria are even dormant, which makes them particularly resistant to antibiotics that are effective only against bacteria in their growth phase. These "persister" cells survive despite increasing doses of antimicrobial agents.[7] In vitro studies have shown that antibiotics can kill bacteria within a biofilm, but the minimum inhibitory concentration (MIC) is 1000 to 1500 times the dose required to kill planktonic bacteria.[2,5]

In addition to resistance against conventional antibiotics, bacterial biofilm also demonstrates resistance to host defenses. The antibody IgG acts against pathogens such as bacteria, fungi, and viruses in the bloodstream by immobilizing the pathogen through agglutination. Against biofilm bacteria, however, IgG is ineffective.[5] Although biofilms cause an intense inflammatory response, the cellular immune response is not effective at destroying a biofilm because neurophils and macrophages responsible for phagocytosis are unable to penetrate the exopolysaccharide and are rendered essentially useless.

Bacteria within a biofilm may spread either as individual cells or as a small clump of detached biofilm. Biofilm bacteria are believed to have the ability to secrete enzymes that degrade the exopolysaccharide matrix and allow individual cells to be dispersed to colonize new surfaces.[7] The dispersed individual cell still retains the

antibiotic resistance characteristic of the parent biofilm, and thus is not susceptible to antibiotics in its planktonic state or as it becomes part of a new biofilm. Bacteria in a biofilm can also spread as a clump when sheared off.[5] For example, forces from blood or other aqueous flow can detach or dislodge a piece of biofilm, causing it to enter the circulation (septic emboli) or spread to another surface. Clumps can also be aerosolized by coughing and subsequently inhaled by another individual, causing spread of bacteria, for example, tuberculosis and Legionnaire disease (**Fig. 2**).

Culturing bacteria for the purpose of identifying the specific bacteria causing an infection is generally only successful for identifying planktonic bacteria, but not bacteria in a biofilm. Because most infections in humans including those in the head and neck are caused by biofilm-associated (sessile) bacteria and not by free-floating (planktonic) bacteria,[5] standard means of culturing a blood or other tissue sample on traditional media is often a fruitless endeavor. Bacteria organized in biofilms grow poorly or not at all on traditional water-based culture media. Environmental microbiologists estimate that only 2% of bacteria occurring in nature can be cultured in the laboratory.[8] Of the 700 known species that comprise the oral flora, only about 50% of these bacteria are culturable.[9] Surgeons are frequently frustrated by the report from the laboratory of "no bacteria found" after submitting a presumed infected implant or an adequate blood or tissue sample for culture. In the past 20 years of performing cultures in a large metropolitan hospital dental service, the authors estimate that less than 10% of culture results have been useful in managing the infection. Knowing that infections are largely caused by biofilms, current research in

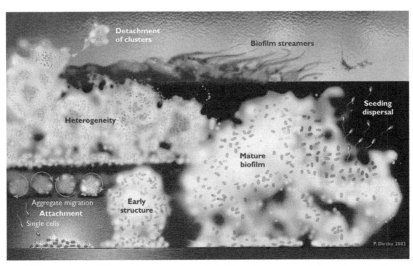

Fig. 2. Conceptual illustration of the heterogeneity of biofilm structure and function. In the foreground, the biofilm life cycle is shown. The midground area shows the heterogeneity in bacterial activity, chemical microenvironments, and microcolony formation. The background shows structural heterogeneities, including streamers and detaching clusters. (*Courtesy of* P. Dirckx; © MSU Center for Biofilm Engineering; with permission.)

microbiology is aimed at identifying the causative organisms by means other than culture and at preventing the establishment of or destroying biofilms by innovative methods.

Infections of the head and neck are among those associated with biofilms. Research in the last decade has demonstrated that otitis media and chronic sinusitis are caused by biofilms even in culture-negative subjects.[10,11] This finding may explain the frequent "reinfections" associated with otitis media and sinusitis as simply exacerbations of persistent biofilm infections. Though rare, necrotizing fasciitis of the head and neck usually begins as soft-tissue trauma that becomes infected by group A *Streptococcus* species, which are known to be able to form biofilms as well.[12]

Many, if not all, infections encountered in the oral and maxillofacial region can also be attributed to biofilms. These infections begin as planktonic "normal oral flora" that become attached to a surface and develop into a biofilm.[5]

DENTAL PLAQUE

One of the most extensively studied biofilms in humans is dental plaque. We learn early in dental education that systemic or topical antibiotics are ineffective in combating tooth decay and periodontitis, and that the mainstay of prevention is the physical removal of bacterial substrates. When one couples the knowledge that dental plaque is a biofilm with the fact that systemic and topical antibiotics do not eradicate biofilm infections, scaling, root planing, and plaque removal

in the practice of preventive dentistry and dental treatment makes perfect sense. However, the biofilm bacteria that cause caries and those that cause periodontal disease are different. Cariogenic biofilms are composed of *Streptococcus mutans* and other acid-producing gram-positive cocci as well as gram-negative bacteria. Plaque originating at the gingival margin is microbially diverse and may include more than 100 species.[13]

CARIES AND APICAL PERIODONTITIS

Immediately after dental prophylaxis, a protein pellicle forms on the surface of the tooth. Oral bacteria beginning with harmless gram-positive cocci such as *Streptococcus salivarius* attach to the tooth surface and organize into a biofilm. A shift in the microbial flora occurs as additional gram-positive bacteria such as *Streptococcus mutans* and gram-negative bacteria ferment dietary carbohydrates and create a more acidic environment, replacing the noncariogenic, acid-intolerant bacteria.[14] *Streptococcus mutans* and other acid-tolerant bacteria such as *Actinomyces* species and lactobacilli flourish. This acidic product of carbohydrate fermentation begins to erode enamel and dentin, allowing for further ingrowth of acid-producing bacteria.

The acidic environment and the presence of the cariogenic biofilm create an intense inflammatory response in the pulp that is experienced as pain by the patient. If the diseased dentin and causative bacteria are not removed, the inflammation will cause necrosis of the pulp. Also, if not removed the bacteria will spread to the pulp and immediately form a biofilm in the pulp chamber and root canal system. In the acute phase of apical periodontitis the apex is sterile, and pain is only experienced as the necrotic pulp causes an inflammatory response at the apex. As the inflammation persists, destruction of the periapical bone occurs and is seen as radiolucency on periapical radiographs. The patient again experiences pain as the biofilm within the canal spreads through the apex and into the periapical bone.

Carious tooth structure and the causative biofilm must be completely excavated to provide symptomatic relief and prevent pulpal spread of the infection. If the biofilm reaches the pulp, removal of the diseased pulp and biofilm is necessary to prevent periapical extension of the infection and possible spread via fascial planes. If the cortex is perforated, spread of the infection can occur into the vestibule or adjacent fascial spaces. Ricucci and Siqueira[15] recently demonstrated the presence of bacterial biofilms in the majority of diseased pulpal and periradicular tissues removed via either apical surgery or extraction. Overall, intraradicular biofilm arrangements were observed in the apical segment of 77% of the root canals (untreated canals: 80%; treated canals: 74%). The prevalence of biofilms in periapical cysts, abscesses, and granulomas was 95%, 83%, and 69.5%, respectively. It is interesting that no correlation was found between biofilms and clinical symptoms or sinus tract presence.

Although extensive research over decades has been performed on the prevention of tooth decay in promising areas such as the development of more effective dentifrices and varnishes, systemic agents, and even vaccinations, the mainstay of tooth decay prevention remains the mechanical removal of the oral biofilm (dental plaque) by professional instrumentation, and regular brushing and flossing.

PERIODONTITIS AND PERI-IMPLANTITIS

Bacteria-laden biofilms have been identified as a major component in periodontal disease and more recently in peri-implantitis, and are now recognized as causing or exacerbating numerous chronic infections.[16]

Extensive evidence has been developed over the years indicating the etiologic role of dental plaque in human oral disease, based on location relative to the gingival margin being divided into supragingival plaque and subgingival plaque. Supragingival plaque is known to be dominated by gram-positive streptococci, which are capable of building up a microorganism community on smooth tooth surfaces and are responsible for dental decay.[17] Subgingival plaque is dominated by gram-negative and anaerobic bacteria, which establish their presence within periodontal pockets and are responsible for marginal periodontitis.[16,18]

The mechanism of plaque biofilm formation on tooth surfaces in the oral cavity is a multistage process. The initial formation of salivary pellicle on the root surface is followed by the adsorption of bacterial cells to the pellicle, which requires specific adhesins, proteins that enable bacterial attachment to surfaces, on the bacterial cell surface. These adhesins are frequently carbohydrate-binding proteins that interact with a complementary receptor on another cell. This process is followed by growth-dependent accumulation by cell-to-cell adhesion to form multilayered cell clusters in a polymeric matrix.[16,17] "The first step is reversible adhesion mediated by electrostatic and hydrophobic forces. The second step is irreversible adhesion caused by a time-dependent shift to a higher state of binding affinity, which involves multiple adhesions on the bacterial surface and polymer matrix."[16,19] The bacterial cells obtain nutrients from the intermicrobial polymer matrix. This matrix is initially populated by *Streptomyces* species. In 1 to 14 days, the plaque changes to one dominated by *Actinomyces* species. This population shift is known as microbial succession. In 2 to 4 weeks the bacterial species become more diverse, with high levels of gram-negative anaerobic filamentous species, and the plaque matures into a biofilm. Supragingival plaque biofilm causes gingivitis, which may proceed to periodontitis, caused by microbes from the subgingival plaque (*Porphyromonas gingivalis*, *Fusobacterium nucleatum*).[9] Dentification using reverse transcription–polymerase chain reaction (RT-PCR) has shown significant differences in the frequencies of the prominent bacteria between supragingival and subgingival plaque.[20]

Biofilm formation on dental implants is similar to that of teeth.[21] Streptococci have been shown to be the predominant initial colonizing microbes on implant material after 4 hours. Anaerobes increased at 48 hours for all implant material studied.[16] Wolf[17] defined the stages of biofilm formation in the oral environment as: association > adhesion > proliferation > microcolonies > biofilm formation > growth maturation. Fürst and colleagues[22] assessed bacterial colonization on oral titanium implants in vivo immediately after implant placement and throughout the first 12 postsurgical weeks. These investigators compared the microbiota at the interproximal subgingival implant surface and adjacent tooth sites, and concluded that bacterial colonization occurred within 30 minutes after placement. The early colonization by streptococci and *Actinomyces* species has been shown to prepare a favorable environment for late colonizers that require more demanding growth conditions (**Fig. 3**). The periodontal pathogens *Porphyromonas*, *Prevotella*, *Capnocytophaga*, and *Fusobacterium* species, which bind to streptococci, are thought to be the causative microorganisms in periodontal infections and peri-implantitis (**Figs. 4 and 5**).[23]

The surface characteristics of metallic bodies such as dental implants play a role in the formation of biofilm because the implants form the base for the bacterial cell to adhere in the oral environment. The surface roughness and surface free energy (SFE) of metal implants influence biofilm formation.[16,24] SFE is the interaction between the forces of cohesion and the forces of adhesion, which determines whether wetting (the spread of a liquid over a surface) occurs. Multiple studies have demonstrated that manipulation of the surface characteristics of implant materials plays a significant role in determining the type and speed of colonization of bacteria on implant and abutment surfaces. Scanning electron microscopy (SEM) was used to evaluate the attachment of oral bacteria on titanium disks with different surface morphologies including smooth, grooved, and rough surfaces.[16,25] The greatest bacterial attachments were observed on rough titanium surfaces, whereas smooth surfaces showed poor attachment. Studies have shown that titanium surfaces with a roughness average (Ra) of 0.088 μm or less and 10-point mean roughness (Rz) of 1.027 μm or less strongly inhibited the accumulation and maturation of plaque. Abutments with such smoothness would inhibit biofilm formation.[25] In other studies hard coatings, such as titanium nitride or zirconium nitride on dental implants, significantly reduced the number of initially adhering bacteria, thereby minimizing plaque biofilm

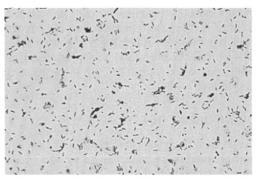

Fig. 4. Heavily colonized gram-negative bacteria around a failing implant (original magnification ×400).

formation and subsequent inflammation of the peri-implant tissues.[26] Both in vitro and in vivo studies have demonstrated that manipulation of surface roughness below 0.2 μm had no increased advantage in reducing bacterial adhesion.

There are several aspects that need to be considered in preventing and managing peri-implantitis. The implant-abutment microgap, abutment material design, and surface characteristics of implant and abutment play significant roles in microbial colonization. The concept of platform switching seems to create space for connective tissue attachment at the implant head, and prevents the bony cupping to the first thread routinely seen with hex head implants. From the evidence, it seems important that the implant surfaces minimize the number of early bacterial colonizers. Rough implant surfaces facilitate more colonization, as the area of adhesion is increased twofold to threefold and the adherent bacteria are sheltered against shear forces in the oral environment.[27]

At present there is little agreement on the management of peri-implantitis once it has begun, and although some innovative claims have been made, this is yet to be followed up with scientific documentation. Attempts at decontaminating the implant with various chemicals and mechanical cleaning have not universally resulted in successful

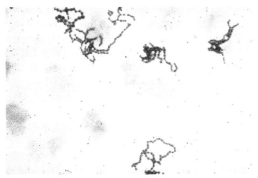

Fig. 3. Sparsely colonized, nonpathogenic gram-positive cocci around a healthy implant (original magnification ×2000).

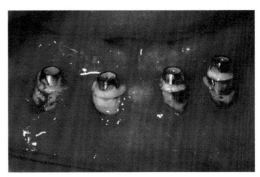

Fig. 5. Significant plaque accumulation around implant abutments.

management. Techniques to graft bone or bone substitutes to exposed threads have usually proved futile. It is therefore imperative that first efforts be directed toward preventing the colonization and biofilm formation, based on the evidence available today.

ODONTOGENIC INFECTIONS

Odontogenic infections are extensions of pulpal or periodontal disease, and may be caused by biofilms that extend beyond the alveolus and often into fascial spaces. Early infections manifest as cellulitis characterized by pain, swelling, and erythema. As the infection progresses, spread into adjacent spaces and abscess formation is possible. Proper treatment of these infections consists of removal of the cause by dental extraction, root canal therapy, periodontal therapy, incision and drainage of abscess formation, or supportive medical therapy including antibiotics. Antibiotics may improve the patient's symptoms by killing the planktonic bacteria that cause a bacteremia, but if the infection is caused by a biofilm, antibiotics alone will not effect a cure.[5] This fact explains why some infections are persistent despite the administration of multiple antibiotics.

BISPHOSPHONATE-RELATED OSTEONECROSIS OF THE JAWS

Bisphosphonate-related osteonecrosis of the jaws (BRONJ) is a devastating side effect of bisphosphonate therapy used for the management of osteoporosis, multiple myeloma, and cancer metastases. BRONJ is defined as persistently exposed bone in the mouth resulting from avascular necrosis secondary to bisphosphonate use (**Fig. 6**).[28] It is usually preceded by local oral trauma such as a dental extraction. Although the etiopathogenesis of osteomyelitis and BRONJ may differ, they share many similarities.

A recent article by Sedghizadeh and colleagues[29] described a prospective study that identified and examined bacterial biofilms microscopically on bone removed due to osteonecrosis in patients taking bisphosphonates. Although the cohort sample was small, the results were striking. All specimens removed and examined by SEM revealed large areas covered with biofilms containing mainly bacteria, but yeasts as well. Common species within the biofilms included *Fusobacterium*, *Actinomyces*, *Streptococcus*, *Staphylococcus*, and *Bacillus* species. Of interest, cross-sectional analysis revealed areas deep within the bone to be colonized with biofilm bacteria, not just the bone exposed to the oral cavity. Other areas of surface bone revealed cavitated resorptive pits filled with multiple species of bacteria. No eukaryotic cells (erythrocytes, leukocytes, osteoclasts) were observed near the resorptive pits, suggesting a direct role of the biofilm in the resorptive process.[29] This finding is clinically relevant, considering the sequestration commonly seen in BRONJ and considering that these patients are taking bisphosphonates specifically to prevent bone resorption.

Treatment of BRONJ is still controversial. Depending on the staging of the BRONJ, many investigators recommend sequestrectomy, debridement, or resection in addition to systemic antibiotics to provide symptomatic relief and possibly prevent spread of the secondary infection.[30–32] Understanding that complex biofilms cover necrotic bone exposed to the oral cavity and even cause resorption may indicate a shift toward more aggressive surgical treatment to relieve symptoms and possibly prevent progression of the disease. In their own experience, the authors have achieved success in promoting the formation of granulation tissue and eventual mucosal coverage of exposed bone only by aggressive debridement of exposed and contaminated bone.

OSTEOMYELITIS

The relationship between osteomyelitis of long bones and bacterial biofilms has been well described. However, very little information has been published on the relationship between biofilms and osteomyelitis of the jaws.

Osteomyelitis of long bones occurs by two methods: hematogenous spread or contiguous focus.[33] Hematogenous osteomyelitis is caused by a seeding of the bone via bacteria in the bloodstream. Contiguous focus osteomyelitis occurs as direct spread of a soft-tissue infection or as a direct inoculation into the bone from local trauma. Infection of orthopedic implants can occur by either hematogenous infection from a bacteremia or contiguous-focus infection from iatrogenic or nosocomial contamination of the implant in the perioperative setting. In the jaws, osteomyelitis occurs as a direct extension of a localized infection. This disease occurs after local trauma such as a dental extraction, a fracture that becomes secondarily infected, periodontal disease, or in association with peri-implantitis. Compromised vascularity and often a compromised host also contribute to the progression of the disease.

The causative microorganisms also differ between osteomyelitis of long bones and osteomyelitis of the jaws. In long bones, *Staphylococcus aureus* and *Staphylococcus epidermidis* are typically the causative microbes. In osteomyelitis of

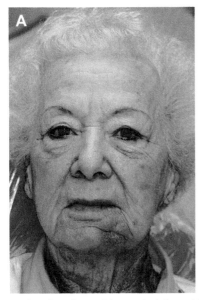

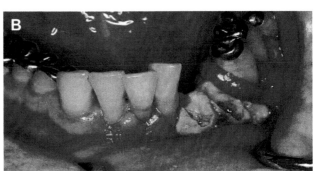

Fig. 6. (*A, B*) Patient with grossly infected bisphosphonate-related osteonecrosis of the jaws.

the jaws, many different microbes contribute to the progression of the disease. Bone exposed to the oral cavity comes in contact with hundreds of species of gram-positive and gram-negative bacteria, both pathogenic and nonpathogenic. Typical bacteria encountered in osteomyelitis of the jaws are *Streptococcus*, *Bacillus*, and *Actinomyces* species, among many others.[34]

Although there are many differences between osteomyelitis of long bones and that of the jaws, both diseases are still caused by bacterial biofilms. Because biofilms are resistant to antibiotic therapy, surgical debridement is still the "necessary" treatment of choice, and antibiotic therapy still has a role as an adjunctive measure (ie, topical oral and systemic antibiotics may kill the planktonic bacteria in the oral cavity and in the bloodstream, and thus improve the patient's symptoms and prevent a bacteremia). Antibiotics may also prevent the formation of new biofilms by killing the planktonic bacteria before they attach to compromised surfaces, for example, necrotic bone.

CURRENT TRENDS

Rather than relying on microbiological culture and sensitivity techniques that have been the standard for decades, new methods of bacterial identification involving microscopy and molecular identification techniques are being used. Confocal scanning laser microscopy allows for very high-resolution identification of bacteria within a biofilm. At very high magnification not only can the individual cells be identified but also the intercellular connections

that allow cell-to-cell communication can be seen.[2,13]

DNA analysis is a very accurate and relatively fast method of bacterial identification. The DNA of a bacterial population is extracted and amplified by PCR.[13] Once amplified, mass spectrometry is used to analyze the ratio of the nucleotides that make up the bacteria's DNA. This means of identification can be performed in a matter of hours compared with several days for culture. Fluorescence in situ hybridization is another method of identifying bacteria.[13] The RNA in bacteria reacts with a chromosomal probe labeled with a fluorophore. By contrast, the RNA of the host does not react, thereby allowing differentiation of host cells from bacterial cells.

Because bacterial biofilms possess multiple means of resistance to antimicrobial agents, a strategy to destroy biofilms must be multifaceted to account for its dynamic and heterogeneous nature. Development of new strategies for killing biofilm bacteria must include targeting "persister" cells deep within the biofilm; this can be achieved either with new or existing drugs or via disruption of gene expression.[7] Disrupting the exopolysaccharide matrix, interrupting the biofilm's means of communication (quorum sensing) and gene transfer that is so vital to biofilm survival, are also important targets of future and ongoing biofilm research.[6,7]

SUMMARY

New information and identification modalities indicate convincingly that the vast majority of infections of the head and neck, and virtually all of those that are encountered in the practice of dentistry and oral and maxillofacial surgery, are caused by bacterial biofilms and not by free-floating, planktonic bacteria. These infections are uniquely resistant to conventional antibiotic therapy. Antibiotics play only a supportive role and cannot be relied upon to cure the infection. Exciting research is under way involving the understanding of the complexities of biofilms. Until new treatment strategies are developed, focusing on the prevention of biofilm formation and disruption of existing biofilms, surgical therapy consisting of removal of diseased tissue and the drainage of pus remains the mainstay of treating these infections.

REFERENCES

1. Parsek MR, Singh PK. Bacterial biofilms: an emerging link to disease pathogenesis. Annu Rev Microbiol 2003;57:677–701.
2. Stewart PS, Costerton JW. Antibiotic resistance of bacteria in biofilms. Lancet 2001;358:135.
3. Lewis K. Riddle of biofilm resistance. Antimicrob Agents Chemother 2001;45:999–1007.
4. Costerton JW, Lewandowski Z, DeBeer D, et al. Biofilms, the customized microniche. J Bacteriol 1994; 176:2137–42.
5. Costerton, JW. Biofilms: definition, clinical implications, chemotherapeutics, effects on periimplantitis. Presentation delivered at AAOMS Dental Implant Conference. Chicago, IL, December 4, 2010.
6. Martin CA, Hoven AD, Cook AM. Therapeutic frontiers: preventing and treating infectious disease by inhibiting bacterial quorum sensing. Eur J Clin Microbiol Infect Dis 2008;27(8):635–42.
7. del Pozo JL, Patel R. The challenge of treating biofilm-associated bacterial infections. Clin Pharmacol Ther 2007;82(2):204–9.
8. Wade W. Unculturable bacteria—the uncharacterized organisms that cause oral infections. J R Soc Med 2002;95(2):81–3.
9. Wilson MJ, Weightman AJ, Wade WG. Applications of molecular ecology in the characterisation of uncultured microorganisms associated with human disease. Rev Med Microbiol 1997;8:91–101.
10. Lee MR, Pawlowski KS, Luong A, et al. Biofilm presence in humans with chronic suppurative otitis media. Otolaryngol Head Neck Surg 2009;141(5):567–71.
11. Hoa M, Syamal M, Schaeffer MA, et al. Biofilms and chronic otitis media: an initial exploration into the role of biofilms in the pathogenesis of chronic otitis media. Am J Otolaryngol 2010;31(4):241–5.
12. Yellon RF. Deep head and neck infections. In: James BS Jr, Shelton CT, editors. Ballenger's otorhinolaryngology head and neck surgery. 17th edition. People's Medical Publishing House; 2009. p. 783–8.
13. Marsh PD. Dental plaque: biological significance of a biofilm and community life-style. J Clin Periodontol 2005;32(Suppl 6):7–15.
14. Marsh PD. Microbiology of dental plaque biofilms and their role in oral health and caries. Dent Clin North Am 2010;54(3):441–54.
15. Ricucci D, Siqueira JF Jr. Biofilms and apical periodontitis: Study of prevalence and association with clinical and histopathologic findings. J Endod 2010;36(8):1277–88.
16. Subramani K, Junq RE, Molenberg A, et al. Biofilm on dental implants: a review of the literature. Int J Oral Maxillofac Implants 2009;24:616–26.
17. Wolf HF. Biofilm—plaque formation on tooth and root surfaces. In: Wolf HF, Rateitschak KH, editors. Periodontology. 3rd edition. Stuttgart (Germany): Thieme; 2005. p. 24.
18. Rosam B, Lamont RJ. Dental plaque formation. Microbes Infect 2000;2:1599–607.
19. Laird WRE, Grant AA. Dental bacterial plaque. Int J Biochem 1983;15:1095–102.
20. Wilson M, O'Connor B, Newman HN. Isolation and identification of bacteria from subgingival plaque with low susceptibility to minocycline. J Antimicrob Chemother 1991;28:71–8.
21. Tanner A, Maiden MF, Lee K, et al. Dental implant infections. Clin Infect Dis 1997;25(Suppl 2):S213–7.
22. Fürst MM, Salvi GE, Lang NP, et al. Bacterial colonization immediately after Installation on oral titanium implants. Clin Oral Implants Res 2007;18:501–8.
23. Mombelli A, Lang NP. Microbial aspects of implant dentistry. Periodontal 2000 1994;4:74–80.
24. Gerber J, Wenaweser J, Heitz-Mayfield L, et al. Comparison of bacterial plaque samples from titanium implant and tooth surfaces by different methods. Clin Oral Implants Res 2006;17:1–7.
25. Rimondini L, Farè S, Brambilla E, et al. The effect of surface roughness on early in vivo plaque colonization on titanium. J Periodontol 1997;68:556–62.
26. Scarano A, Piattelli M, Vrespa G, et al. Bacterial adhesion on titanium nitride-coated and uncoated implants: An in vivo human study. J Oral Implantol 2003;29:80–5.
27. Quirynen M, Van der Mei HC, Bollen CM, et al. The influence of surface-free energy on supra- and subgingival plaque microbiology. J Periodontol 1994;65: 162–7.
28. Reid IR. Osteonecrosis of the jaw—who gets it and why? Bone 2009;44(1):4–10.
29. Sedghizadeh PP, Kumar SKS, Gorur A, et al. Identification of microbial biofilms in osteonecrosis of the jaws secondary to bisphosphonate therapy. J Oral Maxillofac Surg 2008;66(4):767–75.
30. Ruggiero SL, Dodson TB, Assael LA, et al. American Association of Oral and Maxillofacial Surgeons.

American Association of Oral and Maxillofacial Surgeons position paper on bisphosphonate-related osteonecrosis of the jaws—2009 update. J Oral Maxillofac Surg 2009;67(Suppl 5):2–12.

31. Hoefert S, Eufinger H. Relevance of a prolonged preoperative antibiotic regime in the treatment of bisphosphonate-related osteonecrosis of the jaw. J Oral Maxillofac Surg 2011;69(2):362–80.

32. Wilde F, Heufelder M, Winter K, et al. The role of surgical therapy in the management of intravenous bisphosphonates-related osteonecrosis of the jaw. Oral Surg Oral Med Oral Pathol Oral Radiol Endod 2011;111(2):153–63.

33. Brady RA, Leid JG, Calhoun JH, et al. Osteomyelitis and the role of biofilms in chronic infection. FEMS Immunol Med Microbiol 2008;52(1):13–22.

34. Sedghizadeh PP, Kumar SK, Gorur A, et al. Microbial biofilms in osteomyelitis of the jaw and osteonecrosis of the jaw secondary to bisphosphonate therapy. J Am Dent Assoc 2009;140(10):1259–65.

Should Teeth Be Extracted Immediately in the Presence of Acute Infection?

Ankur Johri, DDS, MD, Joseph F. Piecuch, DMD, MD*

KEYWORDS
- Tooth extraction • Infection • Pericoronitis • Third molar

One of the oldest controversial topics in the field of oral and maxillofacial surgery is whether or not to extract teeth immediately in the setting of acute infection. Many dentists and physicians still believe that extraction of teeth in the presence of an acute infection may cause the bacteria to seed into the fascial spaces and cause life-threatening infection in the host.

Although the literature on this topic is dated, the purpose of this article is to review the literature and provide the clinician evidence–based recommendations on extraction of teeth in the setting of an acute infection.

The proponents of delayed extraction recommended postponing the extraction until the infection localizes and the inflammatory response subsides. A large part of this belief stemmed from reports in literature about patients developing severe life-threatening deep fascial space and central nervous system (CNS) infections, or septicemia after extraction of infected teeth. The controversy continued into recent times, with some investigators favoring resolution of infection before tooth removal and others favoring immediate extraction.

Frew,[1] in 1937, based on his personal clinical experience, cautioned against extraction of acutely infected teeth. Frew stated that wisdom teeth with pericoronitis should not be extracted immediately due to risk of inducing cellulitis and death.[1] He suggested that the overlying inflamed operculum provided a "habitat for microorganisms." In his opinion, "meddlesome operative interference" can result in osteomyelitis or cellulitis, resulting in a severe life-threatening infection. Instead, Frew recommended that the patient be placed on antibiotics and that palliative treatment (irrigation around the affected tooth, curettage, excision of the operculum, or removal of the opposing tooth) be performed and the tooth extracted at a later time once the inflammation resolved or the infection formed a walled-off abscess, which can be drained.[2]

Alternatively, Gluck,[3] in 1939, from his clinical experience of approximately 600 patients, found that immediate tooth extraction in the face of acute infection is beneficial. Gluck stressed that immediate extraction avoids putting the patient through continual pain, decreased sleep, and decreased oral intake. Furthermore, removal of the offending tooth removed the source of the infection and provided a path for evacuation of pus through the extraction socket, resulting in faster resolution of the infection. None of his patients suffered from cellulitis or severe life-threatening infections postoperatively. Postoperatively, Gluck's patients did, however, have a transient increase in swelling and trismus, which he attributed to the inflammatory effects of injection of local anesthetic. All his patients, had quick resolution of the infection and of all symptoms after the tooth was extracted.

Wainwright,[4] in 1940, also supported immediate extraction from his clinical experience. He stressed that a necrotic tooth, devoid of blood supply and gangrenous pulp, acts as a "foreign body" and

The authors have nothing to disclose.
Division of Oral and Maxillofacial Surgery, University of Connecticut Health Center, 263 Farmington Avenue, Farmington, CT 06030-1720, USA
* Corresponding author.
E-mail address: piecuch@uchc.edu

Oral Maxillofacial Surg Clin N Am 23 (2011) 507–511
doi:10.1016/j.coms.2011.07.003
1042-3699/11/$ – see front matter © 2011 Elsevier Inc. All rights reserved.

as a "culture medium" and should be removed as quickly as possible. Wainwright suggested that extraction of the tooth re-established the blood supply as well as provided drainage and relieved pain and pressure from the infection.

Haymaker,[5] in 1945, presented a retrospective analysis of 28 cases of CNS infections after tooth extraction. These 28 cases were reported from a pool of 125,000 patients—again illustrating the rare occurrence of CNS infections from dental causes. The teeth were carious, symptomatic, infected, or impacted at the time of extraction. One case of subdural empyema, 12 cases of brain abscess, 2 cases of leptomeningitis, 1 case of encephalitis, 11 cases of cavernous sinus thrombosis, and 1 case of transverse myelitis were analyzed. Seventeen cases involved direct extension into the intracranial cavity and 11 cases involved hematogeneous spread. Lower posterior teeth were the major culprits and most likely to cause hematogeneous spread. Upper posterior teeth were more likely to cause direct spread of the infection. Staphylococcus was the most common organism identified in direct spread via fascial spaces. Direct spread usually resulted in osteomyelitis of the greater wing of the sphenoid bone, resulting in penetration into the cranial cavity. Streptococci were the major bacteria causing hematogeneous spread into the cranial cavity. Some infections ascended into the cranial cavity by the pterygoid plexus, resulting in cavernous sinus thrombosis.

Feldman,[6] in his manual of exodontia in 1951, also supported immediate extraction based on his clinical experience. He suggested that incision and drainage of fluctuant lesions at the time of tooth extraction is also an important adjunct, resulting in quicker host recovery.

Hollin and colleagues,[7] in 1967, reported 2 cases of brain abscess and 3 cases of subdural empyema in patients with dental infections. His work was a retrospective analysis of 5 cases of CNS infections of dental origin in a 25-year time period.[7] Four patients had the symptoms develop after tooth extraction and one after restorative treatment of a carious tooth. The onset of symptoms varied from 4 days to 4 weeks after the procedures. The patients presented with symptoms, such as headaches, mental status changes, vision changes, convulsions, hemiparesis, or hemisensory deficits. All patients were febrile and presented with abnormal lumbar puncture findings. In 3 cases, the suppuration was "sterile." In one case, *Micrococcus foetidus* was cultured. In the one other, *Streptococcus viridans* and *Haemophilus parainfluenzae* were cultured. Surgical débridement and antibiotics were used, but 3 patients

recovered and 2 died. In Hollin and colleagues' analysis, posterior teeth are more likely to contribute to intracranial infection. They concluded that although intracranial complications were rare from dental procedures, the mortality rate is high and early recognition of intracranial infection is crucial to successful treatment and recovery. The concept of "sterile abscess" was prevalent decades ago when the isolation of anaerobic bacteria was difficult and uncommon.

In 1965, Kay presented his research into the nature of pericoronitis.[8] The consideration of "predisposing factors" included upper respiratory tract infections, emotional upset, fatigue, and menstruation.

In his second publication, in 1966, Kay suggested that extraction of teeth in a setting of acute infection was safe.[2] In this article, based on the author's thesis, Kay initially described the prevailing "standard treatment" for subacute pericoronitis, which included "warm saline irrigations of the pericoronal space," "drying...of the area," "insertion into the 'pericoronal pouch' of...50 percent trichloroacetic acid," followed by neutralization of the acid with glycerin. Subsequently the patient was to use warm saline mouth rinses every 2 hours, "as hot as can be tolerated without scalding." Kay stated that use of the acid "always ensures immediate pain relief." When he substituted normal saline for the trichloroacetic acid for 152 patients, none noted rapid relief of the pain. Kay also discussed immediate extraction of the opposing tooth or, alternatively, reduction of its cusps. He thought that this would immediately reduce the pain associated with pericoronitis. In a "test series" of 106 patients for whom he withheld treatment of the opposing tooth, the treatment period was prolonged 5.5 days. When the infection was severe, Kay recommended penicillin, which was satisfactory for most patients. This was in the days before development of significant antibiotic resistance. Kay's earlier article stated, "all cultures were sensitive to penicillin."[8]

Kay performed a trial of 56 patients with "acute" severe pericoronitis, for whom he performed the "standard treatment" as for subacute conditions and 48 (86%) deteriorated significantly. The other 8 resolved without antibiotics but required multiple appointments for treatment, between 8 and 12 visits. Kay considered extraction of the third molar the final solution to pericoronitis but only after the "standard treatments" controlled the infection. The general opinion of the day was as follows. "There is common assent on the advisability of deferring extraction until the symptoms of acute infection have abated, to preclude the putative risk of osteomyelitis."[2] His study (of 1781 patients) also showed that the percentage of dry sockets was almost the same whether the teeth were removed immediately or delayed (even up to 10 weeks). Prior to this time, many thought that early extraction induced a high rate of dry socket.

Subsequently, Kay studied the effects of penicillin on the development of alveolar osteitis (AO).[2] He performed an initial pilot study, a retrospective analysis of 28 patients with pericoronitis for whom immediate extraction was performed. In this patient pool, 20 patients (71%) suffered from postoperative dry socket. In his analysis, the incidence of dry sockets was decreased by using preoperative antibiotics (penicillin G), given intramuscularly 0.5 hour before extraction. Only 2 (8%) of 25 patients treated in this way developed AO. In the same article Kay reported on his "main survey" of 2265 patients. His "control group" of 1341 patients with third molar extraction without antibiotics developed a 24% incidence of AO. A group of 301 patients treated with local anesthesia and a single preoperative dose of intramuscular penicillin developed AO 3.6% of the time. Another group of 623 patients treated under general anesthesia with preoperative antibiotics continued for 3 days and developed AO 2.6% of the time.

The opponents to this notion of resolution of infection before extraction recommend immediate extraction of the offending teeth, regardless of presence of infection, because it results in faster resolution of the infection, quicker recovery of the host, and prevention of potential mortality from these infections.

In 1951, Krogh[9] performed a retrospective study of 3127 patients. Over a 5-year period, he extracted the infected teeth immediately.[9] Typical signs and symptoms preoperatively were aching tooth, extraoral swelling, trismus, and pus in tooth socket. Extraction of teeth in his patients was performed despite any presence of comorbid conditions in the host. Incision and drainage as needed along with the tooth extraction were performed and drains were placed if necessary. The majority of these teeth (91%) were extracted using general anesthesia. Postoperatively, his complication rate was 3% (most of which were minor complications, such as dry socket and postoperative abscesses requiring incision and drainage). None of Krogh's patients developed osteomyelitis or septicemia. None of his patients died. His conclusion was that extraction of infected teeth, and of teeth with acute pericoronitis, as soon as possible results in fewer overall complications than in patients whose extractions were delayed.[9] According to Krogh, by removing the tooth, the nidus of infection is eliminated from the host, preventing extension of the localized infection into the fascial spaces.

Hall and colleagues[10] in 1968 evaluated the temporal relationship between the time of tooth extraction and the resolution of cellulitis in a randomized controlled prospective trial. A total of 350 patients with dental cellulitis were randomly assigned to 2 treatment groups. One group had their teeth extracted on day 1 versus the second group, who were placed on antibiotics and had delayed extraction of their teeth on day 4. The majority of the patients had the procedure performed under local anesthesia, but 6% of the patients required general anesthesia. Incision and drainage and/or systemic antibiotics were also given if deemed necessary by the clinician and the same criteria were used for both groups. The immediate extraction group had faster reduction of pain than the control group. Also the size of the swelling and the oral temperature of the patient also decreased more rapidly in the immediate extraction group. Patients in the delayed extraction group had twice the need for incision and drainage, which, if needed, was also twice as likely to be extraoral than intraoral. Neither group exhibited any intracranial or life-threatening complications. Hall and colleagues' study showed no ill effects or spread of the infection to deeper spaces from immediate extraction of infected teeth. Their conclusion was that immediate extraction of teeth is a safe and effective procedure.

Rud,[11] in 1970, performed a retrospective analysis of removal of 988 impacted lower third molars with acute pericoronitis from 1952 to 1967. A total of 94% of his patients had surgery under local anesthesia. The majority of these teeth with acute pericoronitis were partially impacted (85%) and penicillin was not used in majority of his patients (88%). Postoperatively, there were no instances of osteomyelitis, septicemia, cellulitis, or parapharyngeal abscess. Two percent of Rud's patients developed a postoperative abscess that required incision and drainage. His conclusion was that delay in extraction of teeth can result in septicemia or osteomyelitis and that early removal of infected third molars is prudent. He also concluded that the isolated case reports of systemic spread of infection resulting in death were likely caused by delay in tooth extraction rather than the extraction procedure itself. He further stressed that atraumatic surgical technique results in quicker host recovery. Furthermore, suturing an infected wound by primary closure postextraction is against surgical principles and should be avoided. Rud also stressed that when systemic symptoms are present, systemic antibiotics (penicillin) should be used. He also demonstrated in his study that local anesthetics in the setting of infection can be safely used and effective for removal of infected teeth.[11]

Martis and Karakakis,[12] in a retrospective study published in 1975, extracted 1376 infected teeth; 327 of these teeth had pre-existing fascial space infections. No serious complications were recorded in this study. One patient had a mild postoperative osteomyelitis, which resolved with penicillin. The conclusion from this study was that infected teeth should be removed as quickly as possible, and that it is a safe procedure.

Martis and colleagues[13] in 1978 published another retrospective study of 720 patients undergoing extraction of mandibular third molars with acute pericoronitis. Preoperatively, the patients had classic signs of an acute infection: pain (dolor), redness (rubor), swelling (tumor), warmth (calor), and trismus (functio laesa). Approximately 72% of these teeth were partially erupted. Five percent of the patients required general anesthesia, whereas the remainder had the extraction performed using local anesthesia. Nineteen percent of the patients required an incision and drainage of the odontogenic abscess at the same time as the tooth extraction. No sutures or local (intrasocket) antibiotics were used. Select patients with pre-existing fascial space infections were given systemic antibiotics postoperatively (either ampicillin or erythromycin). On postoperative follow-up, there were no serious outcomes, such as septicemia, cavernous sinus thrombosis, brain abscesses, or osteomyelitis in this study. Postoperative fascial space infections developed in 1.67% of Martis and colleagues' patients (6 patients with buccal space, 5 patients with submandibular space, and 1 patient with parapharyngeal space). These required subsequent incision and drainage. The investigators attributed these complications to delayed surgical intervention rather than the surgical intervention itself. The conclusion was that extraction of acutely infected/abscessed teeth as early as possible prevents spread of infection into the fascial spaces and thus reduces patient discomfort.

According to the literature review on this topic, the earlier infected teeth are removed from the host, the more favorable the outcome. Furthermore, incision and drainage of a fluctuant abscess, if present at the time of surgery, results in rapid relief and resolution of the infection. Moreover, systemic antibiotics in a host with systemic spread of the infection are also an important adjunct to the overall care of patients. Finally, several investigators have shown in their clinical experience that the fear of spreading the infection or causing a life-threatening infection is unjustified and no true cause and effect relationship has been established.

There are, however, some relative indications to delay tooth extraction. Although none of these is an absolute contraindications, prudent clinicians must keep them in mind before performing surgery. These include efficacy of the local anesthetic and comorbid medical conditions, such as diabetes or coagulopathies.

Optimization of a patient's medical condition results in more successful outcomes after major surgery. In minor dentoalveolar surgery, these medical considerations are relative, not absolute, indications for delaying tooth extraction. Nonetheless, it is still crucial to eliminate the source of the infection (ie, the offending tooth) as soon as possible.

In Krogh's article, he describes extracting teeth without delay even in his severely medically ill patients. In his retrospective study, there were no adverse outcomes of extracting infected teeth in patients who were medically ill.[9] Moreover, in an immunocompromised patient, it may be prudent to remove the nidus of infection as soon as possible.

SUMMARY

As seen in this review of the topic, the controversy has been settled for several decades, yet the purpose of the article is to review the evidence on both sides of this question, because concerns arise from time to time, particularly from general dentists and physicians unfamiliar with the oral and maxillofacial surgery literature. The earliest literature—articles before the antibiotic era—considered immediate (at the time of initial diagnosis) extraction to be dangerous. These articles presented primarily the lowest level (level IV) evidence, expert opinion based on personal experience. Later articles suggesting that early extraction did not lead to serious infection or to CNS spread also had lower levels of evidence (level III), retrospective uncontrolled case series. Only the article by Hall and colleagues[10] provided strong evidence (level Ib) in the form of a prospective randomized controlled trial, finding that delaying extraction led to more severe infection, which required more extensive surgery. Currently, most surgeons understand that a combination of surgical extraction and antibiotics can be curative and that watchful waiting, even with antibiotics, is no longer acceptable.

Based on this review of the literature, the recommendation is to extract infected teeth as soon as safely possible, given a patient's overall medical condition. The longer a necrotic tooth remains, the more likely it is to cause a fascial space infection, with greater morbidity and possible mortality. Early extraction, along with incision and drainage, and antibiotics as indicated, hastens recovery. Reports of serious CNS spread of infection after tooth extraction are rare, and a causal relationship between extraction and spread of infection has not been established. Therefore, the belief that extracting infected teeth may cause life-threatening infection is unsubstantiated.

REFERENCES

1. Frew AL. Acute oral infections—when not to extract teeth. J Am Dent Assoc 1937;24:440.
2. Kay LW. Investigations into the nature of pericoronitis—II. Br J Oral Surg 1966;4:52–78.
3. Gluck B. The advisability of immediate extraction in cases of swellings. Dental Items Interest 1939;61:225.
4. Wainwright J. Anesthesia and immediate extraction in the presence of swellings of the jaws. Dental Items Interest 1940;62:849.
5. Haymaker W. Fatal infections of the central nervous system and meninges after tooth extraction, with analysis of 28 cases. Am J Orthod (Oral Surg Section) 1945;31:117.
6. Feldman, MH. A manual of exodontia. 1951. p. 204.
7. Hollin SA, Hayashi H, Gross SD. Intracranial abscesses of odontogenic origin. Oral Surg 1970;23: 277–86.
8. Kay LW. Investigations into the nature of pericoronitis. Br J Oral Surg 1965;3:188–205.
9. Krogh HW. Extraction of teeth in the presence of acute infections. J Oral Surg 1951;9:136–51.
10. Hall HD, Gunter JW, Jamison HC, et al. Effect of time of extraction on resolution of odontogenic cellulitis. J Am Dent Assoc 1968;77:626–31.
11. Rud J. Removal of impacted lower third molars with acute pericoronitis and necrotizing gingivitis. Br J Oral Surg 1970;7:153–60.
12. Martis CS, Karakakis DT. Extractions in the presence of acute infections. J Dent Res 1975;54:59–61.
13. Martis CS, Karabouta I, Lazaridis N. Extraction of impacted mandibular wisdom teeth in the presence of acute infection. Int J Oral Surg 1978;7: 541–8.

Should We Wait for Development of an Abscess Before We Perform Incision and Drainage?

Rabie M. Shanti, DMD, MD, Shahid R. Aziz, DMD, MD*

KEYWORDS
- Abscess • Incision • Drainage • Deep neck infections

Surgical procedures consist of a series of acts repeated in a set precise manner. Disease progression, anatomic variations, and misdiagnosis, however, can place surgeons in unfamiliar situations where a surgeon has to rely on personal experience, surgical principles, and learned adages to successfully carry out a procedure. Examples of such adages include the following: "the key is exposure"; "measure twice and cut once"; "all bleeding eventually stops"; and "if in doubt explore." One adage that has successfully endured the test of time is "never let the sun go down on undrained pus." The latter axiom is taught and emphasized regularly in oral and maxillofacial surgery with regard to the management of deep neck infections. Deep neck infections are infections (either abscess or cellulitis) that are within the potential spaces and fascial planes of the head and neck. The majority of these infections are of odontogenic origin. The source of deep neck infections is known in 30% to 90% of cases, with 52% of known sources of odontogenic origin.[1–5] More than half of these severe odontogenic infections are caused by anaerobic bacteria.[6] Deep neck infections should not be ignored, and no surgeon should underestimate the necessity of appropriate and timely treatment of deep neck infections due to the serious and potentially life-threatening nature of these infections. These infections possess the ability to spread along the fascial spaces of the head and neck, resulting in life-threatening complications, such as airway obstruction, sepsis, mediastinitis, pericarditis, brain abscess (**Fig. 1**), empyema, pneumonia, carotid artery erosion, and jugular vein thrombosis.[7] The most common of these grave complications is upper airway obstruction.[7]

Treatment options for deep neck infections vary from immediate incision and drainage to instituting a trial of intravenous antibiotics; however, confusion regarding which is the most appropriate mode of therapy has risen as a result of imperfect diagnostic measures (ie, clinical examination and radiographic assessment). Traditional algorithms were based on the presence or absence of an abscess. In short, if a localized, fluctuant swelling indicative of an abscess could be appreciated on clinical examination, the patient underwent surgical drainage, applying the surgical adage, "never let the sun go down on undrained pus."[7] Likewise, if a diffuse, indurated swelling indicative of cellulitis was appreciated on clinical examination, the patient received only antibiotics. This approach was based more on opinion unsupported by facts.

The deep neck infection that has generated a greatest amount of debate with regard to immediate incision and drainage versus intravenous antibiotic therapy is the pediatric retropharyngeal abscess. Infections involving the retropharyngeal

Department of Oral and Maxillofacial Surgery, University of Medicine and Dentistry of New Jersey, 110 Bergen Street, Room B-854, Newark, NJ 07103-2400, USA
* Corresponding author.
E-mail address: azizsr@umdnj.edu

Oral Maxillofacial Surg Clin N Am 23 (2011) 513–518
doi:10.1016/j.coms.2011.07.004
1042-3699/11/$ – see front matter © 2011 Elsevier Inc. All rights reserved.

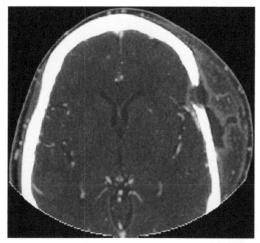

Fig. 1. Brain abscess originating from the deep temporal space secondary to dental disease. (*Courtesy of Maano Milles, DDS, Newark, NJ.*)

space (**Fig. 2**) are ominous, because this potential space extends from the skull base to the superior mediastinum and is also able to impinge directly on the airway. In 1997, a poll of members of the

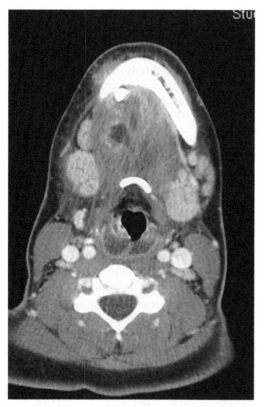

Fig. 2. Contrast-enhanced CT scan of a ring-enhancing retropharyngeal abscess with a smooth contour of the abscess wall. Note the presence of a ring-enhancing abscess in the right submandibular space. (*Courtesy of Vincent B. Ziccardi, DDS, MD, Newark, NJ.*)

American Society of Pediatric Otolaryngology attempted to determine standard practices of the membership of the society in managing retropharyngeal abscesses in children.[8] Of the 138 respondents, which represented 77.5% of the total membership of the society at the time, 51% thought that in 20% to 40% of the cases retropharyngeal abscesses resolved with intravenous antibiotics alone, whereas 13% thought that 60% to 100% of the cases resolved with intravenous antibiotics alone. Furthermore, 22% of the respondents thought that retropharyngeal abscesses would never resolve with intravenous antibiotics alone. Because of concern over the false-positive rate of contrast-enhanced CT in evaluating these infections, and due to the difficulty of accessing the retropharyngeal space, today there are many recommendations primarily in the otolaryngologic literature in support of only using intravenous antibiotic therapy for the management of retropharyngeal abscesses in clinically stable patients.[7,8] Therefore, a dilemma exists as to whether immediate surgical drainage is indicated in all deep neck infections or whether surgical drainage should be reserved until a discrete abscess is formed. Because no current standard of care has been established for the treatment of deep neck infections, this article applies the concepts of evidence-based dentistry to provide readers with the scientific evidence to determine whether all deep neck infections should undergo incision and drainage, or if surgical drainage should be reserved only for infections in the abscess stage.[9,10]

PATHOPHYSIOLOGY

No discussion of the treatment of deep neck infections, especially with regard to timing of incision and drainage, would be complete without first reviewing the stages of infection progression. The differentiation between cellulitis and abscess has become an important issue, with some clinicians basing their mode of management of deep neck infections solely on whether the infection is in the cellulitis or abscess stage. Differentiating between cellulitis and abscess is based on duration, pain, size, localization, palpation, presence of pus, degree of seriousness, and type of bacteria (**Table 1**).[11] During the course of an infection, cellulitis is considered the initial phase, with an abscess forming in the later stage of the infection. Cellulitis and abscess are considered both clinical and radiographic diagnoses. Often, the presence of pus is the main clinical observation in distinguishing between the two, and rim-enhancement on contrast-enhanced CT is the main radiographic observation (**Table 2**).

Table 1
General differences between cellulitis and abscess

Characteristic	Cellulitis	Abscess
Duration	Acute	Chronic
Pain	Severe and generalized	Localized
Size	Large	Small
Localization	Diffuse borders	Well circumscribed
Palpation	Dough to indurated	Fluctuant
Presence of pus	No	Yes
Degree of seriousness	Greater	Less
Bacteria	Aerobic	Anaerobic

Data from Peterson LJ. Principles of management and prevention of odontogenic infections. In: Peterson LJ, Ellis E, Hupp JR, et al, editors. Contemporary oral and maxillofacial surgery. 4th edition. St Louis (MO): Mosby; 2003.

HISTORICAL VIEWS

Since Ludwig[12,13] in 1836 first described 5 cases of a "gangrenous inflammatory induration of the connective tissue of the neck," extensive dispute has been fostered on the appropriate evaluation and management of deep neck infections. For instance, traditional management algorithms were based on the presence or absence of an abscess. The following are a few sample excerpts in opposition to surgical drainage of deep neck infections in the cellulitis stage:

- "Incision and drainage into an unlocalized cellulitis in an erroneous search for pus can disrupt the physiologic barriers and cause diffusion and extension of the infection."[14]
- "Premature incision into an unlocalized cellulitis in an ill-conceived search for pus can disrupt the normal physiologic barriers and cause further diffusion and extension of infection…in the absence of pus, all treatment should be directed toward localizing the infection."[15]
- "It is often difficult to establish whether there is a cellulitis or an abscess. Premature incision into a cellulitis may disrupt the normal barriers and cause further spread of the infection."[16]
- "Early stage infections that initially appear as a cellulitis with soft doughy, diffuse swelling do not respond to incision and drainage procedures."[17]
- "The prerequisites for successful management of deep neck infections include proper

diagnosis and treatment, emphasizing control of the airway, effective antibiotic therapy, and timely surgical intervention…those patients who fail to respond to antibiotic therapy or who progress rapidly require surgical intervention."[18]

Therefore, avoiding surgical drainage of infections in the cellulitis stage was initially prompted by fear of further spread of the infection. Moreover, avoiding unnecessary surgery, and its complications, including anesthetic morbidity and mortality, neurovascular damage, and scarring, motivates surgeons to reserve drainage only for infections in the abscess stage.

The literature also includes recommendations for surgical drainage for all deep neck infections irrespective of the stage of the infection. The following excerpts highlight this opinion:

- "When a case fulfils the criteria prerequisite to a diagnosis of Ludwig's angina, immediate surgical drainage is indicated…fluctuation and pus will develop in about 50 per cent of the cases but only after a matter of days. While one waits, he is exposing his patient to the grave complications here mentioned."[19]
- "To carry out the premise of early treatment, incision and drainage of extraoral abscesses must be performed before the amount of tissue destruction and suppuration is sufficient to be detected by palpation…by prompt treatment, the site of evacuation can be determined cosmetically; the patient is saved discomfort and the possibility of further complications is reduced greatly."[20]

CLINICAL EXAMINATION

Patients with deep neck infections often present with some, but not all, of the following signs and symptoms: fever, dysphagia, odynophagia, floor of mouth elevation, malaise, trismus, toxic appearance, stiff neck, pooling of saliva, stridor, change in vocal quality (hot potato voice), neck swelling, and cervical lymphadenopathy. Patients can also present with worsening of snoring or frank obstructive sleep apnea.[21] Additionally, the clinical presentation is dependent on the involved anatomic spaces. For instance, patients with lateral pharyngeal space infections may present with Horner syndrome (miosis, ptosis, and anhidrosis) as a result of involvement of the cervical sympathetic chain located within the posterior compartment of the lateral pharyngeal space. Mayor and colleagues[3,4] showed that the most common presentation of

Table 2
Contrast-enhanced CT characteristics of cellulitis and abscess

Cellulitis	Abscess
Soft tissue swelling	Soft tissue swelling
Enhancement of involved muscles	Enhancement of involved muscles
Obliterated fat planes	Obliterated fat planes
	Peripheral rim enhancement

deep neck infections was odynophagia in 84% of patients; after that, dysphagia occurred in 71% of patients, followed by fever (68%), neck pain (55%), neck swelling (45%), trismus (39%), and lastly respiratory distress, occurring in 10% of patients with deep neck infections.

In a landmark study by Flynn and colleagues,[6] the accuracy of clinical assessment of deep neck infections was investigated. In this study the accuracy of clinical examination, defined as the frequency of a test's correctly diagnosing the presence or absence of a disease in identifying a drainable collection, was measured at 63%. Other studies have reported a sensitivity of 28% and specificity of 92% in clinically diagnosing an abscess.[7] Additionally, in this cohort the sensitivity of clinical examination, which is the ability of clinical examination to correctly identify the presence

of drainable collection when pus was truly present, was 55%. Furthermore, clinical examination was also shown to have a specificity of 73% in identifying the absence of a drainable collection. Flynn and colleagues[6] also showed that abscess defined by the presence of pus is underestimated, with pus present in the majority (76%) of deep neck infections of odontogenic origin at the time of surgical drainage. These results indicate that clinical assessment underpredicts the presence of an abscess, but if an abscess is diagnosed, then there is a high probability of finding pus on surgical incision and drainage.[7]

DIAGNOSTIC IMAGING

Diagnostic imaging techniques used to evaluate odontogenic infections include plain radiographs, ultrasound, CT, and MRI. Diagnostic imaging plays a central role in the management of patients with deep neck infections. Plain film radiographs are commonly used to diagnose pathologic conditions of odontogenic origin (eg, caries, periapical pathology, and periodontitis). Classically, lateral views of the cervical soft tissues were used to determine the patency of the airway. The lateral view of the cervical soft tissues may be helpful in the treatment of submandibular, parapharyngeal, or retropharyngeal spaces that can cause airway compromise. Contrast-enhanced CT is considered the most accurate and widely used imaging modality in the evaluation of deep neck infections. Early

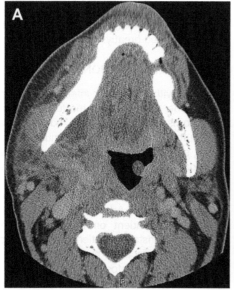 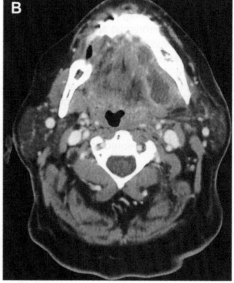

Fig. 3. (*A*) Non-contrast enhanced CT, soft tissue window showing nonenhancing hypodensity in the right pterygomandibular space. (*B*) Contrast-enhanced CT demonstrating a ring-enhancing collection in the left submandibular space.

reports on the accuracy of contrast-enhanced CT scans in diagnosing deep neck infections were favorable, with published reports of 100% accuracy.[22] These studies were, however, nonblinded. In recent studies that reviewed at least 30 patients each, the false-positive rate of contrast-enhanced CT evaluating deep neck abscesses ranged from 11.8% to 25%.[23] The accuracy of CT scans in distinguishing between cellulitis and abscess has generated much of the debate today about the mode of therapy.[24,25] A limitation of most of these studies was a small sample size.[26,27] This has led some to advocate intravenous antibiotics alone for deep neck infections, due to the absence of a surgically drainable collection. In essence, this false-positive rate has led some investigators to recommend intravenous antibiotics alone for the management of deep neck infections. The CT criteria used to differentiate cellulitis from abscess are shown in **Table 2** and illustrated in **Fig. 3**.

In a study by Kirse and Roberson,[21] ring enhancement and irregularity (scalloping) of the collection wall (**Fig. 4**) were analyzed for their value in predicting the presence of pus. This study evaluated contrast-enhanced CT scans of 62 patients. The sensitivity of ring-enhancement was 89%, but its specificity was 0% in this series. Irregularity (scalloping) of the abscess wall, however, was found a more useful predictor of the presence of pus, with a sensitivity of 64% and specificity of 82%. The investigators concluded that pus can be present before scalloping is present, but when scalloping is present pus is almost always found. Based on these data, it can be inferred that the presence of scalloping of the abscess wall is a late development in abscess progression.

The literature also clearly demonstrates that the combination of clinical examination and contrast-enhanced CT have the strongest accuracy, sensitivity, and specificity in diagnosing deep neck infections and in identifying a drainable collection.[28]

SUMMARY

This article has attempted to provide readers with an evidence-based approach to the management of deep neck infections. The aforementioned literature shows that clinical assessment of deep neck infections is not exact, generally underestimating suppuration.[7] The presence or absence of pus is not predicted by any clinical factor, such as preadmission antibiotics, white blood cell count, and duration of swelling.[6,29] The only nonradiographic variable, however, that has been associated with cellulitis is the later identification of Peptostreptococci in culture. Furthermore, contrast-enhanced CT is the preferred technique for imaging of these infections. The combination of clinical assessment and contrast-enhanced CT is the most accurate approach for evaluating these infections. Priority in the care of a patient with a deep neck infection should always be on airway security irrespective of the stage of the infection (cellulitis or abscess). Today, there is no universal agreement on issues, such as optimal timing for surgical drainage and the duration of antibiotic therapy for the management of deep neck infections. The differential diagnosis between cellulitis and abscess is not as critical of an issue in management of these infections. Recent multivariate analysis by Flynn and colleagues[29] indicated that the presence or absence of pus at surgical drainage did not have a statistically significant effect on length of hospital stay. Clinicians must acknowledge limitations in the accuracy in the clinical and radiographic examinations of deep neck infections with regard to differentiation cellulitis from pus. According to the current literature, deep neck infections that can be accurately identified in the cellulitis stage in a clinically stable patient can be successfully treated with intravenous antibiotics alone. If an abscess is suspected, however, management should include planning for immediate surgical drainage. Therefore, it is the authors' opinion that the majority of deep neck infections diagnosed as cellulitis are in actuality abscesses. Instituting a trial of intravenous antibiotics in very clinically stable patients when both clinical and contrast-enhanced CT assessments indicate the infection is in a cellulitis stage is also supported in the current literature.

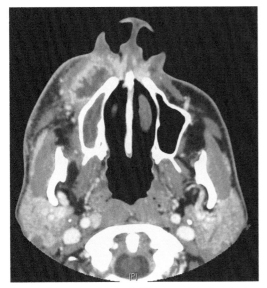

Fig. 4. Contrast-enhanced CT scan of a focal, ring-enhancing infraorbital abscess with an irregular (scalloped) contour of the abscess wall.

REFERENCES

1. Patterson HC, Kelly JH, Stroone M. Ludwig's angina: an update. Laryngoscope 1982;92:370.
2. Bottin R, Marioni G, Rinaldi R, et al. Deep neck infection: a present day complication. A retrospective review of 83 cases (1998-2001). Eur Arch Otorhinolaryngol 2003;260:576.
3. Mayor GP, Milan JM, Martinez-Vidal A. Is conservative treatment of deep neck space infections appropriate? Head Neck 2001;23:126.
4. Osborn TM, Assael LA, Bell RB. Deep space neck infection: principles of surgical management. Oral Maxillofac Surg Clin North Am 2008;20:353.
5. Huang TT, Liu TC, Chen PR, et al. Deep neck infection: analysis of 185 cases. Head Neck 2004; 26:854.
6. Flynn TR, Shanti RM, Levi MH, et al. Severe odontogenic infections, part 1: prospective report. J Oral Maxillofac Surg 2006;64:1093.
7. Courtney MJ, Miteff A, Mahadevan M. Management of pediatric lateral neck infections: does the adage "...never let the sun go down on undrained pus..." hold true? Int J Pediatr Otorhinolaryngol 2007;71:95.
8. Lalakea M, Messner AH. Retropharyngeal abscess management in children: current practices. Otolaryngol Head Neck Surg 1999;121:398–405.
9. Niederman R, Leitch J. "Know what" and "know how" knowledge creation in clinical practice. J Dent Res 2006;85:296.
10. Niederman R, Richards D. Evidence-based dentistry: concepts and implementation. J Am Coll Dent 2005; 72:37.
11. Peterson LJ. Principles of management and prevention of odontogenic infections. In: Peterson LJ, Ellis E, Hupp JR, et al, editors. Contemporary oral and maxillofacial surgery. 4th edition. St Louis (MO): Mosby; 2003. p. 344–66.
12. Ludwig D. [No title]. Med Cor-Bl d Wurttemb Aerztl Ver 1836;6:21–5.
13. Ludwig TK. Angina: a surgical approach based on anatomical and pathological criteria. Ann Otol Rhinol Laryngol 1947;56:937.
14. Moose SM. Acute infections of the oral cavity. In: Kruger GO, editor. Textbook of oral surgery. 3rd edition. St Louis (MO): CV Mosby Co; 1968. p. 166–90.
15. Chow AW, Roser SM, Brady FA. Orofacial odontogenic infections. Ann Intern Med 1978;88:392.
16. Heimdahl A, Nord CE. Orofacial infections of odontogenic origin. Scand J Infect Dis Suppl 1983;39:86.
17. Peterson LJ. Principles of management and prevention of odontogenic infections. In: Peterson LJ, Ellis E, Hupp JR, et al, editors. Contemporary oral and maxillofacial surgery. 2nd edition. St Louis (MO): Mosby; 1993. p. 409–35.
18. Marra S, Hotaling AJ. Deep neck infections. Am J Otol 1996;17:287.
19. Williams AC. Ludwig's angina. Surg Gynecol Obstet 1940;70:140.
20. Laskin DM. Anatomic considerations in diagnosis and treatment of odontogenic infections. J Am Dent Assoc 1964;69:308.
21. Kirse DJ, Roberson DW. Surgical management of retropharyngeal space infections in children. Laryngoscope 2001;111:1413.
22. Endicott JN, Nelson RJ, Saraceno CA. Diagnosis and management decision in infection of the deep fascial spaces of the head and neck utilizing computerized tomography. Laryngoscope 1982;92:630.
23. McClay JE, Murray AD, Booth T. Intravenous antibiotic therapy for deep neck abscesses defined by computerized tomography. Arch Otolaryngol Head Neck Surg 2003;129:1207.
24. Boucher C, Darion D, Fisch C. Retropharyngeal abscesses: a clinical and radiographic correlation. J Otolaryngol 1999;28:134–57.
25. Glasier CM, Stark JE, Jacobs RF, et al. CT and ultrasound imaging of retropharyngeal abscesses in children. Am J Neuroradiol 1992;13:1191–5.
26. Vural C, Gungor A, Comerci S. Accuracy of computerized tomography in deep neck infections in the pediatric population. Am J Otolaryngol 2003;24:143–8.
27. Holt RG, McManus K, Newman RK, et al. Computed tomography in the diagnosis of deep-neck infections. Arch Otolaryngol 1982;108:693–6.
28. Miller WD, Furst IM, Sandor G, et al. A prospective, blinded comparison of clinical examination and computed tomography in deep neck infections. Laryngoscope 1999;109:1873.
29. Flynn TR, Shanti RM, Hayes C. Severe odontogenic infections, part 2: prospective outcomes study. J Oral Maxillofac Surg 2006;64:1104–13.

What are the Antibiotics of Choice for Odontogenic Infections, and How Long Should the Treatment Course Last?

Thomas R. Flynn, DMD

KEYWORDS

- Antibiotics • Odontogenic infection • Treatment course

In view of the constantly changing antibiotic sensitivity patterns of orofacial pathogens and anecdotal reports of treatment failures in orofacial odontogenic infections (OI), oral and maxillofacial surgeons (OMS) must continually make clinical decisions on the choice of empiric antibiotic therapy in the face of uncertainty. In addition, we must decide on the duration of antibiotic treatment empirically, knowing that patients commonly do not complete the prescribed antibiotic course, usually without adverse effect.

Therefore, OMS need updated answers to these 2 questions:

1. What are the empiric antibiotics of choice for OI?
2. How long should the treatment course last?

The first question is the more complex. A contemporary double-blind, randomized controlled clinical trial comparing all of the relevant antibiotics in a large, multicenter, North American population of patients with well-defined OI, combined with appropriate surgical treatments, would be ideal. A similar study of the duration of the antibiotic treatment course, with its long-term effects on selection for antibiotic-resistant bacteria, would provide the answer to the second question. However, such studies do not exist.

Laboratory studies of the antibiotic sensitivities of a large number of pathogens from OI are informative, but they cannot account for the effects of surgical treatment, bacterial interactions, and immune response in the clinical situation.

The OMS must take into account the potential morbidities of the antibiotic and surgical treatments, plus their economic costs, before making the antibiotic prescription.

This article is an attempt to answer these questions with a systematic review of the currently available scientific literature on this multifaceted topic.

MATERIALS AND METHODS
Formulation of the Questions

As the introduction to this article indicates, this broad topic must be broken down into multiple answerable questions, using the PICO format: P = patients; I = intervention(s); C = controls; O = outcomes. Those questions are:

1. In patients with orofacial OI (ie, an OI presenting with swelling going beyond the alveolar process into soft tissue), does administration of 1 antibiotic, compared with another antibiotic or no antibiotic, result in: (a) faster resolution, (b) less morbidity from the infection or the treatment,

The author has nothing to disclose.
1055 Waverly Drive, Reno, NV 89519, USA
E-mail address: thomasrflynndmd@gmail.com

Oral Maxillofacial Surg Clin N Am 23 (2011) 519–536
doi:10.1016/j.coms.2011.07.005
1042-3699/11/$ – see front matter © 2011 Elsevier Inc. All rights reserved.

oralmaxsurgery.theclinics.com

(c) less selection for antibiotic-resistant organisms, or (d) less expense?
2. In patients with OI, does administration of an antibiotic for a 4-day or shorter course, compared with a 5-day or longer course, result in: (a) faster resolution, (b) less morbidity from the infection or the treatment, (c) less selection for antibiotic-resistant organisms, or (d) less expense?

These 2 questions indicate that there are 4 possible significant outcomes that may be measured, and various studies may focus on only some of them. The formulation of a comprehensive answer to these questions also must take into account whether surgical treatment was combined with the antibiotic course, and whether a control (ie, no antibiotic and/or surgery alone) was used in the study design.

There are 2 categories of study that may shed light on the first question. In vitro studies report antibiotic sensitivity testing of bacterial strains cultured from specimens sampled from clinical infections. They measure only the comparative effectiveness of various antibiotics against individual strains of bacteria that may or may not be present in a given clinical infection. In vivo studies that measure the comparative clinical success of various empirically administered antibiotics more closely simulate the clinical situation posed by the first question. Both in vitro and in vivo studies are evaluated, albeit separately, and the clinical studies are given greater weight than the laboratory studies.

Hypotheses

The hypotheses of this systematic review are:

1. Administration of narrow-spectrum antibiotics, such as penicillin, azithromycin, or clindamycin, combined with appropriate surgical treatment, results in equal or better clinical outcomes than broader-spectrum antibiotics or no antibiotic, as measured by time to resolution, morbidity, selection for antibiotic-resistant strains, and expense.
2. Laboratory studies of the antibiotic sensitivities of pathogens in OI indicate that no one antibiotic is effective in all cases.
3. Antibiotic courses of 4 days or less, combined with appropriate surgical treatment, result in equal or better clinical outcomes, as measured by time to resolution, morbidity, selection for antibiotic-resistant strains, and expense.

Search Methodology

Before this review was initiated, the PubMed database, DARE (Database of Abstracts of Reviews of Effects), and the Controlled Trials Register of the Cochrane Library were searched for the period from their inception to December 27, 2010. The term "antibacterial agent" with a subtopic of "therapeutic use", with limitations of human studies and published in English, and application of "review articles" as a publication-type limit, were used to locate systematic reviews on the topic.

To identify relevant clinical trials, these databases were searched from their inception to December 27, 2010. The Specialized Register of Clinical Trials of the Cochrane Oral Health Group was also searched in the same manner. Because of the continually changing nature of bacterial resistance to antibiotics, the laboratory studies of antibiotic sensitivity patterns were limited to those published since January 1, 2000. The strategy for all searches is documented in **Box 1**.

The titles of articles found by these search methods were examined and all potentially relevant articles were selected for review of their abstracts, if available, or the entire article. The reference lists of these articles were also reviewed, and possibly relevant articles were also obtained. In addition, the author's list of references was also reviewed for such articles. All of the articles thus identified were read and evaluated for possible inclusion in this study.

Selection Criteria

The following criteria were used to include or exclude articles from this systematic review:

1. Target population: patients presenting with an oral, facial, or cervical infected swelling of odontogenic origin
2. Interventions: systemically administered antibiotics, local surgical measures, such as incision and drainage, tooth extraction, endodontic therapy, or gingival curettage, and observation
3. Outcome measures: time to a clinical end point, such as resolution of fever, drainage, or swelling, return to work, hospital discharge, or significant symptom relief; morbidity or death caused by the disease or the treatment; selection of antibiotic-resistant strains; and the cost of care
4. Types of studies:
   a. Clinical studies of antibiotic treatments: controlled clinical trials comparing the effectiveness of 2 or more antibiotics, possibly with a negative control (no antibiotic)
   b. Laboratory studies of the comparative antibiotic sensitivity of bacterial strains cultured from odontogenic orofacial infections; because of changing antibiotic resistance patterns over time, only laboratory studies

---

Box 1
Search strategy

Database

MEDLINE (1966 to present)

Search Engine

PubMed

Search Terms

Each search included 1 or more of the search terms and the limits activated

For Clinical Trials

"Periapical Diseases"[Majr] AND "Periapical Diseases/drug therapy"[Majr]

(("anti-bacterial agents"[MeSH Terms] OR ("anti-bacterial"[All Fields] AND "agents" [All Fields]) OR "anti-bacterial agents"[All Fields]) OR "antibiotic"[All Fields] OR "anti-bacterial agents"[Pharmacologic Action]) AND ("bacterial infections"[MeSH Terms] OR ("bacterial"[All Fields] AND "infections" [All Fields]) OR "bacterial infections"[All Fields] OR ("bacterial"[All Fields] AND "infection"[All Fields]) OR "bacterial infection" [All Fields]) AND ("mouth diseases"[MeSH Terms] OR ("mouth"[All Fields] AND "diseases"[All Fields]) OR "mouth diseases"[All Fields]))

"Soft Tissue Infections/drug therapy"[Majr]

("Abscess"[Mesh] OR "Periapical Abscess" [Mesh] OR "Retropharyngeal Abscess"[Mesh] OR "Periodontal Abscess"[Mesh]) AND ("Anti-Bacterial Agents"[Mesh] OR "Anti-Bacterial Agents/therapeutic use"[Mesh])

For Laboratory Studies

(("microbial sensitivity tests"[MeSH Terms] OR ("microbial"[All Fields] AND "sensitivity"[All Fields] AND "tests"[All Fields]) OR "microbial sensitivity tests"[All Fields]) AND ("mouth diseases"[MeSH Terms] OR ("mouth"[All Fields] AND "diseases"[All Fields]) OR "mouth diseases"[All Fields]))

Limits Activated

For Clinical Trials

Humans, Clinical Trial, Meta-Analysis, Practice Guideline, Randomized Controlled Trial

For Laboratory Studies

Humans, published in the last 10 years

---

published between 2000 and 2010 were included

c. Clinical studies of the duration of antibiotic treatment courses: controlled clinical trials

of orofacial OIs comparing 4 days or less with 5 days or more of antibiotic treatment, with or without surgical therapy.

Exclusion Criteria

Clinical studies were excluded for the following reasons, with examples:

1. Population: OI limited to the periodontium or the periapical region; non-OIs; mixed-cause head and neck infections without separate reporting of odontogenic cases
2. Study type: case series or reports, review articles
3. Inappropriate outcome measure: pain relief alone as an outcome measure
4. Controls: lack of clearly stated control or comparison group in clinical studies
5. Randomization: nonrandomized trials
6. Language: articles written in languages other than English.

Laboratory studies were excluded for the following reasons, with examples:

1. Population: OI limited to the periodontium or the periapical region; non-OIs; mixed-cause head and neck infections without separate reporting of odontogenic cases
2. Antibiotics: studies that did not report sensitivities to a penicillin and to clindamycin
3. Bacteria: studies that did not report on both viridans group *Streptococci* and oral anaerobes
4. Sensitivity standards: studies that did not use the National Committee for Clinical Laboratory Standards (NCCLS)/Clinical and Laboratory Standards Institute breakpoints for minimum inhibitory concentration, where available
5. Publication date: studies published before January 1, 2001
6. Language: articles written in languages other than English.

Assessment of Methodological Quality

The clinical studies were amenable to an assessment of the likelihood of the introduction of bias. The quality assessment scale adapted from Jadad and colleagues[1] by Matthews and colleagues[2] was used to assign a numerical quality score, from 0 to 5. It is described fully in **Table 1**. The criteria on which each included article were assessed include randomization, blinding or double-blinding (as appropriate to the study design), and a description of withdrawals and dropouts. The highest possible quality score was 5.

In 1998, the US Food and Drug Administration (FDA) issued guidelines for the development of

Table 1
Jadad quality scale

Question	Answer	Points
1. Was the study described as randomized?	No	0
	Yes	1
	Yes, and the method was described and appropriate	2
	Yes, and the method was inappropriate	0
2. Was the study described as double-blind?	No	0
	Yes	1
	Yes, and the method of double-blinding was described	2
3. Was there a description of withdrawals and dropouts?	No	0
	Yes	1
Total possible score		5

Adapted from Jadad AR, Moore RA, Carroll D, et al. Assessing the quality of reports of randomized clinical trials: is blinding necessary? Control Clin Trials 1996;17(1):1–12; with permission.

antimicrobial drugs for the treatment of complicated skin and soft tissue infections.[3] The 7 guidelines state that such studies should include infections in areas predisposed to polymicrobial infections (eg, the oral cavity); provide clear inclusion, exclusion, and outcome definitions; provide a detailed clinical description of the patients; consider the primary outcome measure to be clinical cure; provide culture data in at least 70% of patients; stratify the analysis of outcomes by surgical intervention, and by clinical cure with evidence of bacterial eradication. The number of these 7 criteria that each included study met was recorded, as an additional measure of quality.

The quality of laboratory studies was assessed by the number of strains per case. The number of strains isolated in the study was divided by the number of patients to calculate the number of strains per case. This statistic was used as a measure of the quality of the microbiologic methods used, based on the assumption that better methods would result in a greater number of bacterial strains isolated in each case.

Data Extraction

Pertinent information was extracted from each clinical study, including study design, sample size, patient characteristics, eligibility criteria, antibiotic regimen, surgical interventions allowed, controls and study groups, outcome measures and results. Similar data from laboratory-based studies were extracted, as appropriate, including antibiotics tested, geographic location, and sensitivity to 80% and to 90% of all strains of all species isolated.

Costs of Oral Antibiotics

The retail cost an uninsured patient would pay for a 1-week prescription for commonly prescribed antibiotics for OIs was obtained from a large pharmacy chain in the Boston area. The cost of a given prescription was divided by the cost of a standard amoxicillin prescription to produce the amoxicillin cost ratio, to provide a numeric means of comparing antibiotic costs.

RESULTS

In the search for review articles, 40 potentially relevant review articles were found, and after evaluation, 3 review articles were selected for discussion in this article. In the preliminary search for relevant studies, 1003 articles potentially relevant to any of the 3 study questions were found. There were 772 articles potentially relevant to antibiotic treatments in OI, 228 articles potentially relevant to antibiotic sensitivity in OI, and 3 trials of antibiotic treatment course duration. Some trials reported both on comparative antibiotic treatments and on bacterial sensitivities. However, none of these met the criteria for inclusion as laboratory studies. After evaluation, 23 clinical trials of antibiotic treatments in OI, 18 laboratory studies of antibiotic sensitivity from OI, and 3 trials of antibiotic treatment course duration were selected for detailed review. The articles that were excluded after detailed review are listed in **Table 2**, with their exclusion criteria.[4–31]

CLINICAL TRIALS OF ANTIBIOTICS

Eight studies met the selection criteria for clinical trials; they are listed in **Table 3**,[32–40] along with selected characteristics. These 8 studies included 488 patients, with a mean of 61 ± 29 (standard deviation [SD]) and a range of 19 to 106 patients per study. The mean quality assessment scale was 2.6 ± 1.3 (range 1–5). The studies are listed in **Table 3** in decreasing order of the power × quality score, which is the number of patients multiplied by the quality assessment scale, with a mean of 150 ± 78 and a range of 38 to 245. The 8 studies met a mean of 4.1 ± 1.1 of the 7 FDA antimicrobial drug development guidelines, with a range of 3 to 6.

A penicillin was either the intervention or comparator antibiotic in all studies. Penicillin V orally was used in 3 studies; penicillin G intramuscularly and amoxicillin/clavulanate were used in 2 studies each, whereas ampicillin and amoxicillin were used in 1 study each. Other antibiotics tested, with the number of trials listed in parentheses, were: clindamycin (2), lincomycin (1), cephalexin (1), metronidazole (1), ornidazole (1), and moxifloxacin (1).

Only 1 study used a nonantibiotic control, consisting of surgery alone. Surgery, consisting of incision and drainage, tooth extraction, or root canal therapy, possibly in combination, was used in all of the studies as an adjunctive treatment in all of the study groups. Only 1 study used hospitalized patients.[32] Intravenous moxifloxacin and amoxicillin/clavulanate (available intravenously in Europe) were compared. All patients received extraoral, with or without intraoral, incision and drainage, or tooth extraction.

None of the 8 studies found a statistically significant difference in clinical cure rate, as defined by the individual study.

There was only 1 study that reported a statistically significant difference between treatment groups. In a randomized, nonblinded trial comparing amoxicillin/clavulanate with penicillin, a significantly lower pain level on days 2 and 3 of treatment was found in the amoxicillin/clavulanate group. There was no difference in clinical cure, which was observed in all patients by day 7.[36]

Nearly significant differences were found in a few other studies. In a randomized, nonblinded trial comparing amoxicillin, cephalexin, and surgery alone, both antibiotic groups had a shorter time to clinical cure, 4.5 days versus 4.7 days versus 6.2 days for amoxicillin, cephalexin, and surgery alone, respectively.[38] In a randomized, operator-blinded study comparing ornidazole and penicillin, there were significantly fewer days with pain in the ornidazole group and more treatment failures in the penicillin group (nearly statistically significant.)[39] However, in this study, 4 of the 60 patients, 2 each in the ornidazole and the penicillin

groups, received no surgery; there was no adjustment for the multiple statistical tests used.

LABORATORY STUDIES

Four studies reported in 6 publications met the selection criteria for laboratory studies of antibiotic sensitivity.[40–45] Two of these studies reported separate portions of their data in 2 separate publications.[41,42,44,45] Thus, 5 articles and 1 letter are included in **Table 4**. These 4 studies included 280 patients, with a mean of 70 ± 28 (SD) and a range of 37 to 94 patients per study. The mean number of strains per case was 3.9 ± 1.3, with a range of 2.4 to 5.5. These studies are listed in **Table 4** in decreasing order of strains per case, which roughly corresponds to the date of publication, with the more recent studies reporting more strains per case.

All of the studies tested the antibiotic sensitivities of the isolated aerobic and anaerobic strains to penicillin or ampicillin, a β-lactam/β-lactamase inhibitor combination, clindamycin, and a fluoroquinolone. Some studies included other antibiotics, including doxycycline, minocycline, erythromycin, various cephalosporins, and impenem. Either levofloxacin or moxifloxacin were the fluoroquinolones tested, and the β-lactam/β-lactamase inhibitor combinations were either amoxicillin/clavulanate or ampicillin/sulbactam. In 1 study, metronidazole was tested against obligate anaerobes only, and gentamicin was tested only against viridans group *Streptococci*.

The overall results of these studies indicate that no one antibiotic is likely to be effective in vitro against all strains of all species, although Blandino and colleagues[40] stated that the combination of penicillin and metronidazole would have been effective against all strains of all species, consistent with the clinical strategy of using 1 antibiotic highly effective against the oral *Streptococci* and another for the oral anaerobes. In 2 of the 4 studies, amoxicillin/clavulanate or impenem was effective against 90% or more of all strains of all species.[40,43] In 1 study, levofloxacin, cefoxitin, and cefotaxime were also effective against 90% or more of all strains of all species.[40] In 3 of the 4 studies, a β-lactam/β-lactamase inhibitor combination was effective against 80% of all strains of all species.[40–43] In 2 of the 4 studies, clindamycin, a cephalosporin, imipenem, or a fluoroquinolone was effective against 80% of all strains of all species.[43–45]

The most recent study[44,45] found that no antibiotic was even 80% effective against all strains of all species isolated, although imipenem and cephalosporins were not tested. In the clinical portion of

Table 2
Excluded articles

Reference	Reason for Exclusion
Clinical Trials	
Adriaenssen CF. Comparison of the efficacy, safety and tolerability of azithromycin and co-amoxiclav in the treatment of acute periapical abscesses. J Int Med Res 1998;26(5):257–65[4]	2
Benson EA. Antibiotics in surgical treatment of septic lesions. Lancet 1970;1(7658):1233[5]	3
Brennan MT, Runyon MS, Batts JJ, et al. Odontogenic signs and symptoms as predictors of odontogenic infection: a clinical trial. J Am Dent Assoc 2006;137(1):62–6[6]	4
Chien JW, Kucia ML, Salata RA. Use of linezolid, an oxazolidinone, in the treatment of multidrug-resistant gram-positive bacterial infections. Clin Infect Dis 2000;30(1):146–51[7]	2
Daramola OO, Flanagan CE, Maisel RH, et al. Diagnosis and treatment of deep neck space abscesses. Otolaryngol Head Neck Surg 2009;141(1):123–30[8]	2
Ellison SJ. The role of phenoxymethylpenicillin, amoxicillin, metronidazole and clindamycin in the management of acute dentoalveolar abscesses—a review. Br Dent J 2009;206(7):357–62[9]	3
Fouad AF, Rivera EM, Walton RE. Penicillin as a supplement in resolving the localized acute apical abscess. Oral Surg Oral Med Oral Pathol Oral Radiol Endod 1996;81(5):590–5[10]	2
Hanna Jr CB. Cefadroxil in the management of facial cellulitis of odontogenic origin. Oral Surg Oral Med Oral Pathol 1991;71(4):496–8[11]	3
Herrera D, Roldán S, O'Connor A, et al. The periodontal abscess (II). Short-term clinical and microbiological efficacy of 2 systemic antibiotic regimes. J Clin Periodontol 2000;27(6):395–404[12]	2
Hood FJ. The place of metronidazole in the treatment of acute oro-facial infection. J Antimicrob Chemother 1978;4(Suppl C):71–3[13]	3
Lo Bue AM, Sammartino R, Chisari G, et al. Efficacy of azithromycin compared with spiramycin in the treatment of odontogenic infections. J Antimicrob Chemother 1993;31(Suppl E):119–27[14]	2
Matijević S, Lazić Z, Nonković Z [Clinical efficacy of ampicillin in treatment of acute odontogenic abscess]. Vojnosanit Pregl 2009;66(2):123–8[15]	1
Ozbek C, Aygenc E, Unsal E, et al. Peritonsillar abscess: a comparison of outpatient i.m. clindamycin and inpatient i.v. ampicillin/sulbactam following needle aspiration. Ear Nose Throat J 2005;84(6):366–8[16]	2
Panosetti E. Phlegmonous and abscess-forming ENT infections: comparative efficacy of ceftriaxone versus amoxicillin-clavulanic acid. ORL J Otorhinolaryngol Relat Spec 1992;54(2):95–9[17]	2
Rambo WM, Del Bene VE, Burkey LG, et al. Comparison of moxalactam with the combination of clindamycin and an aminoglycoside in the treatment of common surgical infections. Rev Infect Dis 1982;4(Suppl):S683–7[18]	2

Laboratory Studies

Al-Nawas B, Maeurer M. Severe versus local odontogenic bacterial infections: comparison of microbial isolates. Eur Surg Res 2008;40(2):220–4. [Epub 2007 Nov 12][20]   5

Eckert AW, Maurer P, Wilhelms D, et al [Bacterial spectra and antibiotics in odontogenic infections. Renaissance of the penicillins?]. Mund Kiefer Gesichtschir 2005;9(6):377–83[21]   1

Gorbach SL, Gilmore WC, Jacobus NV, et al. Microbiology and antibiotic resistance in odontogenic infections. Ann Otol Rhinol Laryngol Suppl 1991;154:40–2[22]   6

Heimdahl A, von Konow L, Satoh T, et al. Clinical appearance of orofacial infections of odontogenic origin in relation to microbiological findings. J Clin Microbiol 1985;22(2):299–302[23]   6

Kuriyama T, Absi EG, Williams DW, et al. An outcome audit of the treatment of acute dentoalveolar infection: impact of penicillin resistance. Br Dent J 2005;198(12):759–63[24]   7

Kuriyama T, Karasawa T, Nakagawa K, et al. Antimicrobial susceptibility of major pathogens of orofacial odontogenic infections to 11 beta-lactam antibiotics. Oral Microbiol Immunol 2002;17(5):285–9[25]   8

Kuriyama T, Karasawa T, Williams DW, et al. An increased prevalence of {beta}-lactamase-positive isolates in Japanese patients with dentoalveolar infection. J Antimicrob Chemother 2006;58(3):708–9[26]   8

Kuriyama T, Nakagawa K, Karasawa T, et al. Past administration of beta-lactam antibiotics and increase in the emergence of beta-lactamase-producing bacteria in patients with orofacial odontogenic infections. Oral Surg Oral Med Oral Pathol Oral Radiol Endod 2000;89(2): 186–92[27]   7

Kuriyama T, Williams DW, Yanagisawa M, et al. Antimicrobial susceptibility of 800 anaerobic isolates from patients with dentoalveolar infection to 13 oral antibiotics. Oral Microbiol Immunol 2007;22(4):285–8[28]   2

Lo Bue AM, Sammartino R, Chisari G, et al. Efficacy of azithromycin compared with spiramycin in the treatment of odontogenic infections. J Antimicrob Chemother 1993;31(Suppl E):119–27[14]   2

Müller HP, Holderrieth S, Burkhardt U, et al. In vitro antimicrobial susceptibility of oral strains of Actinobacillus actinomycetemcomitans to 7 antibiotics. J Clin Periodontol 2002;29(8):736–42[29]   2

Sixou JL, Magaud C, Jolivet-Gougeon A, et al. Evaluation of the mandibular third molar pericoronitis flora and its susceptibility to different antibiotics prescribed in France. J Clin Microbiol 2003;41(12):5794–7[30]   2

Duration of Antibiotic Therapy

Martin MV, Longman LP, Hill JB, et al. Acute dentoalveolar infections: an investigation of the duration of antibiotic therapy. Br Dent J 1997;183(4):135–7[31]   3

1, Language other than English; 2, population not OI; 3, type not randomized clinical trial; 4, type not a comparison of antibiotics or duration of antibiotic therapy; 5, sensitivities not reported for all isolates; 6, publication date before 2001; 7, design not prospective; 8, sensitivities do not include at least penicillin and clindamycin.

Table 3
Included clinical trials of antibiotics in OI

Reference	Year	N	Quality Assessment Scale[a]	Power × Quality Score	Number of FDA Guidelines Met	Intervention Group	Comparator Group	Surgical Control	Significant Difference Between Groups?	Comment
Gilmore et al,[34] 1988	1988	49	5 (2,2,1)	245	6	PCN	CLI	N	N	Only surgery was I&D; ext/RCT performed only after study completion
von Konow and Nord,[39] 1983	1983	60	4 (2,1,1)	240	4	ORN	PCN	N	N	Only surgery was I&D; 2 patients in each group did not receive surgery. Fewer days of pain in ornidazole group (*P*<.05); more failures in PCN group (NSD)
Mangundjaja and Hardjawinata,[37] 1990	1990	106	2 (1,0,1)	212	4	CLI	AMP	N	N	Only surgery was I&D; ext/RCT performed only after study completion. Not all patients were cured by 7 d
Lewis et al,[36] 1993	1993	78	2 (1,0,1)	156	3	AM/CL	PCN	N	N	Surgery was either I&D or ext or RCT. Greater pain reduction at 1–2 d and 2–3 d in amoxicillin/clavulanate group; otherwise NSD in swelling, temperature, lymphadenopathy, or pain

Study	Year		Jadad score			LIN (IM and by mouth)	PCNG (IM and by mouth)			Comments
Davis Jr and Balcom 3rd,[33] 1969	1969	49	3 (1,1,1)	147	3			N	N	9 patients had trauma and fractures, including osteomyelitis
Matijević et al,[38] 2009	2009	90	1 (1,0,0)	90	5	AMOX	CEPH	Y	N	Antibiotic groups had shorter treatment time than surgery alone (not statistically significant)
Ingham et al,[35] 1977	1977	37	2 (1,1,0)	74	3	MET	PCNG (IM once daily)	N	N	Patients received "appropriate surgery when necessary." At 24–48 h, "marked clinical improvement" was noted in all patients
Al-Nawas et al,[32] 2009	2009	19	2 (1,0,1)	38	5	MOXI	AM/CL	N	N	Only study of hospitalized patients, requiring extraoral and/or intraoral I&D. Cure = improving trismus, no pain on palpation, afebrile

Abbreviations: AMP, ampicillin; AM/CL, amoxicillin/clavulanate; AMOX, amoxicillin; CEPH, cephalexin; CLI, clindamycin; ext, extraction; I&D, incision and drainage; IM, intramuscularly; LIN, lincomycin; MET, metronidazole; MOXI, moxifloxacin; N, no; NSD, no significant difference; ORN, ornidazole; PCN, penicillin V; PCNG, penicillin G; RCT, root canal therapy; Y, yes.

a The numbers in parentheses are the components of the Jadad score as in **Table 1** (randomization, blinding, withdrawals/dropouts).

Table 4
Laboratory studies of the antibiotic sensitivity of pathogens in OI

Reference	Year	N	Strains Per Case	Location	Antibiotics Tested	Antibiotics Effective for ≥ 80% of All Strains of All Species	Antibiotics Not Effective for ≥ 80% of All Strains of All Species	Antibiotics Effective for ≥ 90% of All Strains of All Species	Comment
Warnke et al,[45] 2008	2008	94	5.50	Germany	PCN, CLI, AM/CL, MOXI, DOXY	None	PCN, CLI, AM/CL, MOXI, DOXY	None	MOXI was effective in at least 90% of all strains, except *Clostridium* sp and *Pseudomonas aeruginosa* (1 isolate). Antibiotic + surgery was effective in 98% of all patients
Warnke et al,[44] 2008	2008								Data from this report are combined with the above report
Blandino et al,[40] 2007	2007	56	4.20	Italy	PCN, CLI, AM/CL, ERY, MET^a, LEV, CEFOX, CEFOT, IMI	CLI, AM/CL, LEV, CEFOX, CEFOT, IMI	PCN, ERY, MET	AM/CL, LEV, CEFOX, CEFOT, IMI	MET not tested on aerobic/facultative strains. PCN + MET would have been effective for all strains
Kuriyama et al,[42] 2001	2001	93	3.39	Japan	CLI, AMP, AMP/SUL, ERY, LEV, CEFAZ, CEFOT, CEFMET, IMI, MINO	CLI, AMP/SUL, CEFOT, IMI	AMP, ERY, LEV, CEFAZ, CEFMET, MINO	IMI	GENT was tested only against VGS, with 30% of strains resistant; MET was tested only against obligate anaerobes, with 10% of strains resistant
Kuriyama et al,[41] 2002	2002								Data from this report are combined with the above report
Sobottka et al,[43] 2002	2002	37	2.35	Germany	PCN, CLI, AM/CL, LEV, MOXI, DOXY	AM/CL, MOXI	PCN, CLI, LEV, DOXY	AM/CL	Only AM/CL was effective against all strains of all species

Abbreviations: AMP, ampicillin; AM/CL, amoxicillin/clavulanate; AMP/SUL, ampicillin/sulbactam; CEFAZ, cefazolin; CEFMET, cefmetazole; CEFOT, cefotaxime; CEFOX, cefoxitin; CLI, clindamycin; DOXY, doxycycline; ERY, erythromycin; GENT, gentamicin; IMI, impenem; LEV, levofloxacin; MET, metronidazole; MINO, minocycline; MOXI, moxifloxacin; PCN, penicillin.

this study, appropriate surgery alone (36% of cases), or in combination with an antibiotic (64%), resulted in satisfactory recovery in 92 of the 94 cases. In 2 cases (2%), an antibiotic change to cefotaxime was required because of a poor response to penicillin. The choice among no antibiotic, penicillin, or amoxicillin/clavulanate was based on clinical severity. Clindamycin was used in penicillin allergy. The clinical portion of this study was not included among the antibiotic trials, because the patients were not randomly allocated to treatment groups.

The recent in vitro studies of the antibiotic sensitivity of isolates from OIs indicate that there is a trend toward increasing resistance to the commonly used antibiotics, and that newer and broader-spectrum antibiotics have lower resistance rates than older, narrower-spectrum antibiotics. However, even among these studies, there is evidence to indicate that surgical therapy is necessary and often sufficient treatment of orofacial OIs.

DURATION OF ANTIBIOTIC THERAPY

Two studies met the selection criteria for trials of the duration of antibiotic therapy; they are listed in **Table 5**, along with selected characteristics.[46,47] The 2 studies included 101 patients, with a mean of 51 ± 13 (SD) and a range of 41 to 60 patients per study. The mean quality assessment scale, as described in **Table 1**, was 4.5–0.7 (range 4–5). The studies are listed in decreasing order of the power × quality score, which is the number of patients multiplied by the quality assessment scale, with a mean of 225 ± 21 and a range of 210 to 240. Both studies met 3 of the of the 7 FDA antimicrobial drug development guidelines.

Both studies compared short (1–3 days) with long (5–7 days) courses of a penicillin, without the use of a surgery-alone group as a control. All patients received appropriate surgical treatment, consisting of incision and drainage, extraction, or pulpal drainage, possibly in combination. Chardin and colleagues[47] compared amoxicillin 1 g by mouth twice a day for 3 days with the same regimen for 7 days. Lewis and colleagues[46] compared 2 3-g doses of amoxicillin by mouth 8 hours apart with penicillin V 250 mg by mouth 4 times a day. There was no difference in clinical cure at 7 days of treatment between groups in either of the 2 included studies. Neither study used a nonantibiotic control consisting of surgery alone.

Lewis and colleagues[46] observed less swelling at 24 hours after the beginning of treatment in the amoxicillin group, but there was no other difference between groups at any measurement interval

in any of the study parameters (pain, swelling, lymphadenopathy, or temperature). The statistically significant difference in swelling at 24 hours may indicate more rapid antibiotic effectiveness in the amoxicillin group, but there was no statistical adjustment for the multiple tests used. In this study, normalization of the 4 parameters outlined earlier defined clinical cure of the infection, which was achieved at 7 days.

Although the Chardin and colleagues[47] study claimed that a shorter treatment course would result in less selection for the survival of amoxicillin-resistant strains, the difference in carriage of amoxicillin-resistant organisms between the short and long course groups was minimal and nonsignificant at the end of the 30-day observation period.

The 2 included studies found no significant difference in clinical cure at 7 days when either a 1-day to 3-day or a 5-day to 7-day course of antibiotics was used, in combination with appropriate surgery. In 1 study, clinical parameters may have indicated a more rapid decrease of swelling with amoxicillin than penicillin.

Costs of Oral Antibiotics

The retail costs of commonly prescribed antibiotic regimens for OI are listed in **Table 6**. The amoxicillin cost ratio allows numeric comparison of the other antibiotics to the cost of amoxicillin, which is one of the least costly of antibiotics listed. The cost of the 150-mg capsule of generic clindamycin is significantly less than half of the cost of the generic 300-mg capsule. Thus, a prescription for 2 150-mg capsules of generic clindamycin 4 times a day is only 63% of the cost of 1 300-mg capsule 4 times a day for the generic formulation. The brand-name formulation costs even more for the 300-mg capsule.

DISCUSSION

Potential sources of bias in this systematic review include publication bias (unpublished studies were not sought), language bias (only English articles were reviewed), and subjective bias, because only the author reviewed and selected articles. However, language-restricted and language-inclusive meta-analyses do not seem to differ in their estimate of the effectiveness of an intervention.[48] Meta-analysis of the data was not attempted in this review.

Clinical trials that are not randomized or blinded have a greater likelihood of reporting results that favor treatment over control than randomized and blinded ones.[1] It has been shown that inadequate randomization methods can exaggerate the estimated effect of treatment by 41%, and

Table 5
Included trials of the duration of antibiotic therapy

Title/Reference	Year	N	Quality Assessment Scale[a]	Power × Quality Score	Number of FDA Guidelines Met	Intervention Group	Comparator Group	Surgical Control	Significant Difference Between Groups?	Comment
Lewis et al,[46] 1986	1986	60	4 (2,2,0)	240	5	AMOX 3 g every 8 h × 2 doses	PCN 250 mg 4 times a day × 5 d	N	Less swelling at 24 h in AMOX group	No significant difference in pain, swelling, temperature, or lymphadenopathy at day 7
Chardin et al,[47] 2009	2009	41	5 (2,2,1)	210	5	AMOX 1 g twice a day × 3d, then placebo	AMOX 1 g twice a day × 7d	N	N	No difference in carriage of AMOX-resistant Streptococci between groups at 30 d after treatment.

Abbreviations: AMOX, amoxicillin; N, no; PCN, penicillin V.
[a] The numbers in parentheses are the components of the Jadad score as in **Table 1** (randomization, blinding, withdrawals/dropouts).
Data from Jadad AR, Moore RA, Carroll D, et al. Assessing the quality of reports of randomized clinical trials: is blinding necessary? Control Clin Trials 1996;17(1):1–12.

Table 6
Costs of oral antibiotics

Antibiotic	Usual Dose	Usual Interval	Wholesale Cost 2010 ($)	1-Week Retail Cost 2010 ($)	Amoxicillin Cost Ratio
Penicillins					
Amoxicillin	500 mg	8 h	0.37	11.99	1.00
Penicillin V	500 mg	6 h	0.74	12.29	1.03
Augmentin	875 mg	12 h	5.05	51.99	4.34
Augmentin XR	2000 mg	12 h	7.38	108.99	9.09
Dicloxacillin	500 mg	6 h	1.20	25.59	2.13
Cephalosporins (generation)					
Cephalexin Caps (first)	500 mg	6 h	1.23	15.19	1.27
Cefadroxil (first)	500 mg	12 h	3.60	49.49	4.13
Cefuroxime (second)	500 mg	8 h	8.02	84.99	7.09
Cefaclor ER (generic)	500 mg	12 h	4.15	64.59	5.39
Cefdinir (third)	600 mg	24 h	10.22	65.59	5.47
ERYTHROMYCINS					
Erythromycin base	500 mg	6 h	0.30	17.99	1.50
Clarithromycin (Biaxin XL)	500 mg	24 h	5.01	34.69	2.89
Azithromycin (Zithromax)	250 mg	12 h	7.78	120.99	10.09
Telithromycin (Ketek)	800 mg	24 h	11.52	102.99	8.59
Anti-anaerobic					
Clindamycin (generic)	150 mg	6 h	1.19	31.79	2.65
Clindamycin (2 T generic)	300 mg	6 h	2.38	59.99	5.00
Clindamycin (generic)	300 mg	6 h	3.76	87.59	7.31
Metronidazole	500 mg	6 h	0.73	34.49	2.88
OTHER					
Trimethoprim/ sulfamethoxazole	160/800 mg	12 h	0.66	11.99	1.00
Vancomycin	125 mg	6 h	29.10	849.99	70.89
Ciprofloxacin	500 mg	12 h	5.31	13.49	1.13
Moxifloxacin (Avelox)	400 mg	24 h	16.35	138.99	11.59
Doxycycline	100 mg	12 h	1.14	11.99	1.00
Linezolid (Zyvox)	600 mg	12 h	91.97	1322.99	110.34

Notes: Usual doses and intervals are for moderate infections, and are not to be considered prescriptive. Amoxicillin cost ratio = retail cost of antibiotic for 1 week/retail cost of amoxicillin for 1 week.
Courtesy of Aaron Van Dolson, CPhT (Certified Pharmacy Technician).

when the methods of randomization are unclear, the estimate of treatment effect is exaggerated by 30%.[49] Only trials that were described as randomized were included in this review. However, some of the included trials did not further describe their randomization methods, which could exaggerate the estimate of treatment effect.

Jadad and colleagues[1] developed a validated, well-accepted, yet simple scale for evaluating methodological quality of clinical trials based on the grading of 3 parameters: randomization, double- blinding, and description of withdrawals and dropouts. One point is given for each of these parameters if there is a statement that the parameter was used in the study methods. An additional point is added each for randomization and double-blinding, if the method of each was appropriate, and a point is taken away for each of these parameters if the method was inappropriate. Thus, a maximum of 2 points each can be given for randomization and double-blinding, and a maximum of 1 point can be given for a description of withdrawals and dropouts, for a total of 5. The Jadad scale was used in this review.

Double-blinding in studies in which a surgical procedure is involved requires that the evaluator is not the surgeon, and that the evaluator is unaware of whether surgery occurred, and if it did, the nature of the procedure. In assessing randomization, 1 point was awarded if the methods included words such as random, randomly, or randomization. An additional point was awarded if the randomization method was further described and it was appropriate, such as the use of a table of random numbers or computer-generated randomization. The first point was taken away if an inappropriate (predictable) allocation method, such as alternating patients or odd/even medical record numbers, was used. A study was not considered randomized if treatment allocation was stratified by severity, such as minor infections receiving outpatient surgery and oral antibiotics, whereas severe infections were treated with hospital admission, extraoral surgery, and intravenous antibiotics.

The FDA has published guidelines for the development of antimicrobial drugs for the treatment of uncomplicated and complicated skin and skin-structure infections.[3] OIs are considered complicated infections according to these guidelines because of their polymicrobial nature, especially involving anaerobic bacteria. The guidelines include 7 characteristics, listed earlier in the materials section, that antimicrobial trials should show to be considered valid for new antibiotic development. Three criteria (analysis of outcomes stratified by surgical intervention, 70% of patients microbiologically evaluable, and confirmed bacterial eradication at clinical cure) were not consistently met. In 5 of the 8 clinical trials of antibiotics, 70% or more of the subjects were cultured. In 2 studies, the report of outcome (clinical cure) was stratified by surgical intervention. None of the studies reported bacterial eradication by follow-up culture, which is difficult to accomplish when intraoral drainage has been performed. These criteria do not apply to the laboratory studies.

The studies identified in this review did not measure the outcomes of antibiotic morbidity and antibiotic resistance in a comprehensive manner. Antibiotic toxicities, side effects, and drug interactions have been discussed in multiple texts and reviews. The reader is referred to the available literature for more information on those topics, which may be of assistance in the individualized selection of antibiotic for a given patient.

Matthews and colleagues[2] performed a systematic review and meta-analysis of treatments, including antibiotic therapy, for acute apical abscesses with or without swelling. Some of the articles included in that review are also included here. Swelling was a criterion for inclusion in this review. Matthews and colleagues' findings were similar to those of this review: only 1 of the studies reported a significant treatment effect, less pain on day 2 to 3 in the amoxicillin/clavulanate group, compared with penicillin V, but no difference in clinical cure at 7 days. When all studies were combined by meta-analysis, the 95% confidence interval did not exclude the possibility that there was no difference between the intervention and the control antibiotic. Further, these investigators' meta-analysis of 2 studies that included a surgery-only control concluded that there was no significant difference in the number of days to pain resolution between the antibiotic and the surgery-alone groups.

Brennan and colleagues[6] performed a randomized, double-blind clinical trial comparing penicillin V and no antibiotic in preventing OI in patients presenting to a hospital emergency room with toothache. There was no difference in the development of OI in patients receiving penicillin or no antibiotic. On multivariate analysis, the only variables that predicted the development of OI were the presence of a filling or a periapical radiolucency larger than 1.5 mm at the painful tooth. This is high-quality evidence to indicate that the commonly given antibiotic prescription for toothache does not prevent a spreading infection.

In a recent review of the microbiology of periapical abscess, Robertson and Smith[50] noted that unculturable bacteria have been frequently identified in significant proportions from periapical abscesses by using molecular methods to directly identify bacteria in pus specimens by their DNA or RNA. This finding has also been reported in OI.[51,52] Diaz-Torres and colleagues have used molecular methods to identify antibiotic resistance genes in the oral flora.[53] The 4 laboratory studies included in this review all used conventional culturing methods, which is the current standard. In the future, molecular methods are likely to affect our understanding of the flora and antibiotic resistance patterns of OI.

Ellison[9] has reviewed the rational use of penicillin, clindamycin, and metronidazole in dentistry. This historical review, in which the references were selected by the author, comes to the conclusion that these 3 antibiotics should be effective, when combined with the appropriate surgical intervention, when signs of systemic involvement are present, such as fever, tachycardia, swelling, lymphadenopathy, or trismus. Ellison states that surgical treatment alone is effective when systemic signs are absent. He also noted that metronidazole used alone has been shown to be effective in OI when combined with appropriate surgery, even although its spectrum includes only obligate anaerobes.

When systemic signs of infection, such as fever, swelling, lymphadenopathy, or trismus are present, it seems reasonable to prescribe an antibiotic. In 1 study,[38] the time to resolution was shorter when an antibiotic was added to surgery, but this result was not statistically significant.

The recent in vitro studies of the antibiotic sensitivity of isolates from OIs indicate that there is a trend toward increasing resistance to the commonly used antibiotics, and that newer and broader-spectrum antibiotics have lower resistance rates than older, narrower-spectrum antibiotics. However, even among these studies, there is evidence to indicate that surgical therapy is necessary and often sufficient treatment of orofacial OIs.

The results of this systematic review allow us to arrive at a few conclusions.

1. In patients with orofacial OIs receiving appropriate surgical treatment consisting of incision and drainage and/or tooth extraction or root canal therapy, randomized clinical trials comparing 1 antibiotic with another have found no significant difference in the number of patients cured between the intervention and comparator antibiotics.
2. Laboratory studies describing the antibiotic sensitivities of bacterial isolates from orofacial OIs indicate that newer and broader-spectrum antibiotics are more effective in vitro than older, narrower-spectrum antibiotics.
3. In patients with orofacial OIs receiving appropriate surgical treatment consisting of incision and drainage and/or tooth extraction or root canal therapy, randomized clinical trials comparing 3 to 4 days and 7 days of antibiotic therapy have found no significant difference in the number of patients cured between the shorter and the longer course of treatment.

Thus, it seems reasonable to conclude that when combined with appropriate surgery, including incision and drainage, extraction, or root canal therapy, the surgeon's choice of antibiotic should depend on cost and safety, with only minor consideration given to the comparative effectiveness of antibiotics within a given class. A 3-day to 4-day regimen of antibiotic therapy should be adequate in otherwise healthy patients.

Based on this review, the antibiotics of choice for OI are listed in **Table 7**. The choices are

Table 7	
Empiric antibiotics of choice for OIs	
Severity/Penicillin Allergy	**Antibiotics of Choice**
Outpatient	Amoxicillin Clindamycin Azithromycin
Penicillin allergy	Clindamycin Azithromycin Metronidazole Moxifloxacin
Inpatient	Ampicillin/sulbactam Clindamycin Penicillin + metronidazole Ceftriaxone
Penicillin allergy	Clindamycin Moxifloxacin Vancomycin + metronidazole

stratified by severity (inpatient vs outpatient) and by penicillin allergy. Intravenously available antibiotics are listed for inpatient infections.

The β-lactam antibiotics have an excellent safety profile when allergic reaction has been ruled out by a thorough medical history review. The costs of penicillin V and amoxicillin are low and comparable. However, amoxicillin may provide more rapid improvement in pain or swelling, and it is slightly less expensive than penicillin V. Further, compliance with the prescribed antibiotic regimen may be better with amoxicillin because of its longer dosage interval.

In a prospective case series of severe OI requiring hospitalization, Flynn and colleagues found a 21% therapeutic failure rate of intravenous penicillin G in severe, hospitalized cases of OI, and that penicillin-resistant strains were isolated from the infection in 54% of cases.[54,55] Al-Nawas and colleagues[32] found an increased rate of penicillin resistance in hospitalized versus outpatient OI. These findings indicate that it may be prudent to use a β-lactam/β-lactamase inhibitor combination, such as ampicillin/sulbactam as the first-line antibiotic in severe OI requiring hospitalization. This apparent association between antibiotic resistance and virulence in OI warrants further investigation.

In penicillin allergy, clindamycin replaces the β-lactam antibiotics as the drug of choice for safety reasons. Antibiotic-associated colitis (AAC) caused by colonic overgrowth of *Clostridium difficile* is a concern with multiple antibiotics, including clindamycin. However, the demographics of OI do no match those most commonly associated with AAC, which include prolonged hospitalization, abdominal surgery, advanced age, female gender, and multiple comorbidities. In recent years, the diagnosis of AAC has been made easier and faster by the *C difficile* exotoxin assay, and the treatment with either metronidazole or vancomycin orally is generally effective. There is a subset of AAC, fulminant AAC, which manifests as the sudden onset of acute abdomen with high fever and severe leukocytosis. In 1 case series, emergent total colectomy was the only life-saving measure.[56] However, clindamycin does not cross the blood-brain barrier well, which limits its use in OIs that may spread into the central nervous system.

Among the macrolide antibiotics, azithromycin has fewer drug interactions than clarithromycin and erythromycin. Because azithromycin is metabolized by a different pathway than the other macrolides, CYP3A4, the liver microsomal enzyme associated most frequently with drug interactions, is avoided. Therefore, the interactions between the macrolides and statin-type antihyperlipidemic agents, the theophyllines, azole antifungal antibiotics, and warfarin drugs are avoided with azithromycin. Azithromycin has been found effective in 1 clinical study of OI.[57]

Metronidazole has been shown to be as effective as penicillin when used alone in outpatient OIs, when combined with appropriate surgery, even although it kills only anaerobic bacteria.[35] In inpatient infections, the combination of metronidazole with penicillin should be effective against nearly all odontogenic pathogens.[40] This combination crosses the blood-brain barrier.

Moxifloxacin is a fourth-generation fluoroquinolone that is effective against the oral *Streptococci* and anaerobes, including especially *Eikenella corrodens*, which is uniformly resistant to clindamycin. When *E corrodens* has been cultured, moxifloxacin is an excellent antibiotic choice when the initial antibiotic and surgery have not been completely effective. Another advantage of this drug is its excellent absorption and bone penetration when given orally. Moxifloxacin may thus avoid the necessity for a peripherally inserted central catheter in osteomyelitis. It should be avoided in pregnant women and children because of its toxicity to growing cartilage. In adults, Achilles tendonitis has been reported with moxifloxacin.[58] Achilles tendon rupture, leading to death, has occurred with levofloxacin.[59]

Cephalosporins have also been shown to be effective in OI in laboratory studies.[40–42] Ceftriaxone is a third-generation cephalosporin that crosses the blood-brain barrier, unlike most cephalosporins. Ceftriaxone may cause sludging of the bile salts, resulting in pseudocholelithiasis. However, in penicillin allergy, the cephalosporins must be used with caution because of the risk of cross-sensitivity.

A possible alternative antibiotic combination that may be effective in the patient for whom all other antibiotics are contraindicated is vancomycin to cover gram-positive organisms plus metronidazole to cover obligate anaerobes. However, this combination has not been tested for clinical effectiveness in OI.

SUMMARY

The results of this systematic review may allow OMSs to have less concern over the choice of antibiotic prescription in the management of OI. Among the antibiotics commonly used for OI, it seems that no one antibiotic is clearly superior to all others. Antibiotics may therefore be chosen according to cost and safety, with individualized consideration of the patient's medical history. Surgical treatment, consisting of incision and drainage and removal of the odontogenic cause by extraction, endodontic therapy, or other means, is of primary importance.

REFERENCES

1. Jadad AR, Moore RA, Carroll D, et al. Assessing the quality of reports of randomized clinical trials: is blinding necessary? Control Clin Trials 1996;17(1):1–12.
2. Matthews DC, Sutherland S, Basrani B. Emergency management of acute apical abscesses in the permanent dentition: a systematic review of the literature. J Can Dent Assoc 2003;69(10):660 Review.
3. Guidance for industry: uncomplicated and complicated skin and skin structure infections–developing antimicrobial drugs for treatment. US Food and Drug Administration (FDA); 21 July 1998. Available at: http://www.fda.gov/downloads/Drugs/Guidance ComplianceRegulatoryInformation/Guidances/ucm 071185.pdf. Accessed March 15, 2010.
4. Adriaenssen CF. Comparison of the efficacy, safety and tolerability of azithromycin and co-amoxiclav in the treatment of acute periapical abscesses. J Int Med Res 1998;26(5):257–65.
5. Benson EA. Antibiotics in surgical treatment of septic lesions. Lancet 1970;1(7658):1233.
6. Brennan MT, Runyon MS, Batts JJ, et al. Odontogenic signs and symptoms as predictors of odontogenic infection: a clinical trial. J Am Dent Assoc 2006;137(1):62–6.
7. Chien JW, Kucia ML, Salata RA. Use of linezolid, an oxazolidinone, in the treatment of multidrug-resistant

gram-positive bacterial infections. Clin Infect Dis 2000;30(1):146–51.

8. Daramola OO, Flanagan CE, Maisel RH, et al. Diagnosis and treatment of deep neck space abscesses. Otolaryngol Head Neck Surg 2009;141(1):123–30.

9. Ellison SJ. The role of phenoxymethylpenicillin, amoxicillin, metronidazole and clindamycin in the management of acute dentoalveolar abscesses– a review. Br Dent J 2009;206(7):357–62.

10. Fouad AF, Rivera EM, Walton RE. Penicillin as a supplement in resolving the localized acute apical abscess. Oral Surg Oral Med Oral Pathol Oral Radiol Endod 1996;81(5):590–5.

11. Hanna CB Jr. Cefadroxil in the management of facial cellulitis of odontogenic origin. Oral Surg Oral Med Oral Pathol 1991;71(4):496–8.

12. Herrera D, Roldán S, O'Connor A, et al. The periodontal abscess (II). Short-term clinical and microbiological efficacy of 2 systemic antibiotic regimens. J Clin Periodontol 2000;27(6):395–404.

13. Hood FJ. The place of metronidazole in the treatment of acute oro-facial infection. J Antimicrob Chemother 1978;4(Suppl C):71–3.

14. Lo Bue AM, Sammartino R, Chisari G, et al. Efficacy of azithromycin compared with spiramycin in the treatment of odontogenic infections. J Antimicrob Chemother 1993;31(Suppl E):119–27.

15. Matijević S, Lazić Z, Nonković Z. Clinical efficacy of ampicillin in treatment of acute odontogenic abscess. Vojnosanit Pregl 2009;66(2):123–8 [in Serbian].

16. Ozbek C, Aygenc E, Unsal E, et al. Peritonsillar abscess: a comparison of outpatient i.m. clindamycin and inpatient i.v. ampicillin/sulbactam following needle aspiration. Ear Nose Throat J 2005;84(6): 366–8.

17. Panosetti E. Phlegmonous and abscess-forming ENT infections: comparative efficacy of ceftriaxone versus amoxicillin-clavulanic acid. ORL J Otorhinolaryngol Relat Spec 1992;54(2):95–9.

18. Rambo WM, Del Bene VE, Burkey LG, et al. Comparison of moxalactam with the combination of clindamycin and an aminoglycoside in the treatment of common surgical infections. Rev Infect Dis 1982; 4(Suppl):S683–7.

19. Sakaguchi M, Sato S, Ishiyama T, et al. Characterization and management of deep neck infections. Int J Oral Maxillofac Surg 1997;26(2):131–4.

20. Al-Nawas B, Maeurer M. Severe versus local odontogenic bacterial infections: comparison of microbial isolates. Eur Surg Res 2008;40(2):220–4.

21. Eckert AW, Maurer P, Wilhelms D, et al. Bacterial spectra and antibiotics in odontogenic infections. Renaissance of the penicillins?. Mund Kiefer Gesichtschir 2005;9(6):377–83 [in German].

22. Gorbach SL, Gilmore WC, Jacobus NV, et al. Microbiology and antibiotic resistance in odontogenic infections. Ann Otol Rhinol Laryngol Suppl 1991; 154:40–2.

23. Heimdahl A, von Konow L, Satoh T, et al. Clinical appearance of orofacial infections of odontogenic origin in relation to microbiological findings. J Clin Microbiol 1985;22(2):299–302.

24. Kuriyama T, Absi EG, Williams DW, et al. An outcome audit of the treatment of acute dentoalveolar infection: impact of penicillin resistance. Br Dent J 2005;198(12):759–63.

25. Kuriyama T, Karasawa T, Nakagawa K, et al. Antimicrobial susceptibility of major pathogens of orofacial odontogenic infections to 11 beta-lactam antibiotics. Oral Microbiol Immunol 2002;17(5):285–9.

26. Kuriyama T, Karasawa T, Williams DW, et al. An increased prevalence of {beta}-lactamase-positive isolates in Japanese patients with dentoalveolar infection. J Antimicrob Chemother 2006;58(3): 708–9.

27. Kuriyama T, Nakagawa K, Karasawa T, et al. Past administration of beta-lactam antibiotics and increase in the emergence of beta-lactamase-producing bacteria in patients with orofacial odontogenic infections. Oral Surg Oral Med Oral Pathol Oral Radiol Endod 2000;89(2):186–92.

28. Kuriyama T, Williams DW, Yanagisawa M, et al. Antimicrobial susceptibility of 800 anaerobic isolates from patients with dentoalveolar infection to 13 oral antibiotics. Oral Microbiol Immunol 2007;22(4): 285–8.

29. Müller HP, Holderrieth S, Burkhardt U, et al. In vitro antimicrobial susceptibility of oral strains of Actinobacillus actinomycetemcomitans to seven antibiotics. J Clin Periodontol 2002;29(8):736–42.

30. Sixou JL, Magaud C, Jolivet-Gougeon A, et al. Evaluation of the mandibular third molar pericoronitis flora and its susceptibility to different antibiotics prescribed in France. J Clin Microbiol 2003;41(12): 5794–7.

31. Martin MV, Longman LP, Hill JB, et al. Acute dentoalveolar infections: an investigation of the duration of antibiotic therapy. Br Dent J 1997;183(4):135–7.

32. Al-Nawas B, Walter C, Morbach T, et al. Clinical and microbiological efficacy of moxifloxacin versus amoxicillin/clavulanic acid in severe odontogenic abscesses: a pilot study. Eur J Clin Microbiol Infect Dis 2009;28(1):75–82.

33. Davis WM Jr, Balcom JH 3rd. Lincomycin studies of drug absorption and efficacy. An evaluation by double-blind technique in treatment of odontogenic infections. Oral Surg Oral Med Oral Pathol 1969; 27(5):688–96.

34. Gilmore WC, Jacobus NV, Gorbach SL, et al. A prospective double-blind evaluation of penicillin versus clindamycin in the treatment of odontogenic infections. J Oral Maxillofac Surg 1988;46(12): 1065–70.

35. Ingham HR, Hood FJ, Bradnum P, et al. Metronidazole compared with penicillin in the treatment of acute dental infections. Br J Oral Surg 1977;14(3):264–9.

36. Lewis MA, Carmichael F, MacFarlane TW, et al. A randomised trial of co-amoxiclav (Augmentin) versus penicillin V in the treatment of acute dentoalveolar abscess. Br Dent J 1993;175(5):169–74.

37. Mangundjaja S, Hardjawinata K. Clindamycin versus ampicillin in the treatment of odontogenic infections. Clin Ther 1990;12(3):242–9.

38. Matijević S, Lazić Z, Kuljić-Kapulica N, et al. Empirical antimicrobial therapy of acute dentoalveolar abscess. Vojnosanit Pregl 2009;66(7):544–50.

39. von Konow L, Nord CE. Ornidazole compared to phenoxymethylpenicillin in the treatment of orofacial infections. J Antimicrob Chemother 1983;11(3):207–15.

40. Blandino G, Milazzo I, Fazio D, et al. Antimicrobial susceptibility and beta-lactamase production of anaerobic and aerobic bacteria isolated from pus specimens from orofacial infections. J Chemother 2007;19(5):495–9.

41. Kuriyama T, Karasawa T, Nakagawa K, et al. Bacteriology and antimicrobial susceptibility of gram-positive cocci isolated from pus specimens of orofacial odontogenic infections. Oral Microbiol Immunol 2002;17(2):132–5.

42. Kuriyama T, Karasawa T, Nakagawa K, et al. Incidence of beta-lactamase production and antimicrobial susceptibility of anaerobic gram-negative rods isolated from pus specimens of orofacial odontogenic infections. Oral Microbiol Immunol 2001;16(1):10–5.

43. Sobottka I, Cachovan G, Stürenburg E, et al. In vitro activity of moxifloxacin against bacteria isolated from odontogenic abscesses. Antimicrobial Agents Chemother 2002;46(12):4019–21.

44. Warnke PH, Becker ST, Springer IN, et al. Penicillin compared with other advanced broad spectrum antibiotics regarding antibacterial activity against oral pathogens isolated from odontogenic abscesses. J Craniomaxillofac Surg 2008;36(8):462–7.

45. Warnke PH, Becker ST, Springer IN, et al. 'Grandmother penicillin'–not in vogue, but clinically still effective. J Antimicrob Chemother 2008;61(4):960–2.

46. Lewis MA, McGowan DA, MacFarlane TW. Short-course high-dosage amoxycillin in the treatment of acute dento-alveolar abscess. Br Dent J 1986;161(8):299–302.

47. Chardin H, Yasukawa K, Nouacer N, et al. Reduced susceptibility to amoxicillin of oral streptococci following amoxicillin exposure. J Med Microbiol 2009;58(Pt 8):1092–7.

48. Moher D, Pham B, Klassen TP, et al. What contributions do languages other than English make on the results of meta-analyses? J Clin Epidemiol 2000;53(9):964–72.

49. Schulz KF, Chalmers I, Hayes RJ, et al. Empirical evidence of bias: dimensions of methodological quality associated with estimates of treatment effects in controlled trials. JAMA 1995;273:408–12.

50. Robertson D, Smith AJ. The microbiology of the acute dental abscess. J Med Microbiol 2009;58:155–62.

51. Kim Y, Flynn TR, Donoff RB, et al. The gene: the polymerase chain reaction and its clinical application. J Oral Maxillofac Surg 2002;60:808–15.

52. Dymock D, Weightman AJ, Scully C, et al. Molecular analysis of microflora associated with dentoalveolar abscesses. J Clin Microbiol 1996;34(3):537–42.

53. Diaz-Torres ML, Villedieu A, Hunt N, et al. Determining the antibiotic resistance potential of the indigenous oral microbiota of humans using a metagenomic approach. FEMS Microbiol Lett 2006;258(2):257–62.

54. Flynn TR, Shanti RM, Levi MH, et al. Severe odontogenic infections, part 1: prospective report. J Oral Maxillofac Surg 2006;64(7):1093–103.

55. Flynn TR, Shanti RM, Hayes C. Severe odontogenic infections, part 2: prospective outcomes study. J Oral Maxillofac Surg 2006;64(7):1104–13.

56. Morris LL, Villalba MR, Glover JL. Management of pseudomembranous colitis. Am Surg 1994;60(7):548–51.

57. Al-Belasy FA, Hairam AR. The efficacy of azithromycin in the treatment of acute infraorbital space infection. J Oral Maxillofac Surg 2003;61(3):310–6.

58. Burkhardt O, Köhnlein T, Pap T, et al. Recurrent tendinitis after treatment with two different fluoroquinolones. Scand J Infect Dis 2004;36(4):315–6.

59. Gottschalk AW, Bachman JW. Death following bilateral complete Achilles tendon rupture in a patient on fluoroquinolone therapy: a case report. J Med Case Reports 2009;3:1.

Should Prophylactic Antibiotics Be Used for Patients Having Removal of Erupted Teeth?

Daniel M. Laskin, DDS, MS

KEYWORDS

- Prophylactic antibiotics • Erupted tooth • Bacteremia
- Tooth removal • Postextraction infection

The prophylactic use of antibiotics refers to the administration of these agents preoperatively to prevent a postoperative infection. Generally, antibiotics should not be required before the removal of erupted carious or periodontally involved teeth unless a significant risk of postoperative infection is present. Although extraction sockets are considered contaminated wounds, the organisms involved are part of the normal oral flora, and therefore are not a usual source of postextraction infection. However, the decision to use prophylactic antibiotics in noninfected cases should also be based on whether patients have any significant medical risk factors that could adversely affect their humoral and cellular defense mechanisms, and whether any systemic risks are associated with the bacteremia that accompanies tooth extraction. This article discusses the various indications for using prophylactic antibiotics in patients having erupted teeth extracted based on a consideration of these factors.

ERUPTED TEETH IN HEALTHY PATIENTS

Ordinarily prophylactic antibiotics are not indicated in healthy patients without periapical infection who will be having erupted teeth removed. However, the question remains whether patients with existing periapical infection having teeth extracted should be given preoperative antibiotics. Although by definition this practice should be considered therapeutic rather than prophylactic, technically it could be considered prophylactic because it is being used to prevent further spread of an infection that is currently contained within the jaw bone. Under these circumstances, the use of antibiotics should depend on whether the existing periapical infection is acute or chronic. A chronic infection indicates that the body defenses have it contained and antibiotics should not be necessary. However, with an acute periapical infection, the use of antibiotics would depend on whether pus has already formed, which would indicate that the body has controlled the infection, or whether there is still only an osteitis. In the former instance, extraction of the tooth establishes drainage and eliminates the cause, and antibiotics should not be necessary. In the latter instance, the lack of suppuration indicates that the infection has not been contained and antibiotics are probably indicated. However, this hypothesis has never been tested.

Patients may also present with an odontogenic infection that has spread beyond the jaw bone into the adjacent soft tissues. If the result is a vestibular cellulitis, treatment through tooth extraction should be accompanied by antibiotic prophylaxis to prevent further spread of infection. However, if a vestibular abscess is present, tooth extraction and drainage of the abscess should be sufficient. In patients with a fascial space infection, immediate tooth extraction is not crucial, because

Department of Oral and Maxillofacial Surgery VCU School of Dentistry and VCU Medical Center, 521 North 11th Street, PO Box 980566, Richmond, VA 23298-0566, USA
E-mail address: dmlaskin@vcu.edu

Oral Maxillofacial Surg Clin N Am 23 (2011) 537–539
doi:10.1016/j.coms.2011.07.006

oralmaxsurgery.theclinics.com

it will generally not result in drainage of the pus. Therefore, the decision to treat with antibiotics depends on the presence of a cellulitis or an abscess and not whether a tooth will be extracted.

ERUPTED TEETH IN PATIENTS WITH MEDICAL RISK FACTORS

In patients undergoing extraction of erupted teeth, the medical risk factors that may indicate the use of prophylactic antibiotics fall into two categories: those associated with an existing systemic condition that makes patients more susceptible to developing a postoperative infection, and those associated with the consequences of the bacteremia that accompanies tooth extraction.

Systemic Conditions Predisposing to Postoperative Infections

Several conditions can affect the humoral and cellular defense mechanisms that protect the body against infection, theoretically making one more susceptible. These conditions include poorly controlled diabetes; end-stage renal disease and uremia; severe alcoholism; immunocompromising diseases such as HIV, leukemia, lymphoma, and advanced malignancy; and the use of chemotherapeutic agents and other immunosuppressive drugs. Based on this, many clinicians agree that prophylactic antibiotics are indicated in most of these situations.[1–4]

However, this opinion is not supported by the literature. For example, a recent prospective, observer-blinded study on the relationship of glycemic control to the outcome of routine dental extractions in diabetics showed no difference in postextraction healing between well-controlled and poorly controlled people with diabetes.[5] Moreover, studies have also shown that routine extraction is a low-risk procedure for postoperative infection in patients with HIV, particularly when the CD4 count is 200 or greater.[6–8] Investigators have also shown that routine extractions can be performed without prophylactic antibiotics in patients with renal disease who do not have an intravascular access device or an arteriovenous shunt.[9]

In patients on dialysis and who have such an access portal, investigators have suggested that antibiotic prophylaxis may be necessary because of the risk of infection and subsequent bacterial endocarditits.[10] However, the American Heart Association (AHA) does not recommend this in patients without known cardiac risk factors because of the low risk.[11] This advisement is confirmed by two systematic reviews of the literature on the subject, which found no evidence to support the administration of prophylactic antibiotics before routine tooth extraction to prevent indwelling venous catheter infections.[9,12] Similar findings have been reported for cerebrospinal shunts and vascular grafts.[9] The Lockhart and colleagues[9] study also found no indication for prophylactic antibiotics in patients with immunosuppression secondary to cancer or cancer chemotherapy.

Finally, although patients with alcoholic liver disease have reduced reticuloendothelial capacity and altered cell-medicated immune function,[13] studies show that prophylactic antibiotics are not indicated when routine dental extraction is performed.[10]

Consequences of Extraction-Induced Bacteremia

Studies have shown that the incidence of bacteremia after tooth extraction ranges from 43% to 96%, with *Streptococcus viridans* the most commonly involved organism.[14] These bacteremias can persist for as long as an hour after the procedure.[15] In patients with certain forms of heart disease, this has been implicated as potential cause of bacterial endocarditis, and prophylactic antibiotics are commonly used in these patients before teeth are extracted.[11] However, the prominent role of extraction-induced bacteremia in causing bacterial endocarditis was recently questioned,[14] and even the number of indications for prophylactic antibiotics has been reduced in the current AHA guidelines.[11] Moreover, studies have shown that even when prophylactic antibiotics are given, bacteria are still present in the blood stream 1 hour after the procedure[15]; therefore, prophylaxis is not 100% effective. Finally, a Cochrane Database Systematic Review published in 2008 concluded that no evidence shows that penicillin prophylaxis is effective in preventing bacterial endocarditis in patients undergoing invasive dental procedures.[16] However, despite such findings, because of the medicolegal ramifications of noncompliance with published guidelines, the current AHA guidelines should be followed in patients undergoing routine dental extractions.

The use of prophylactic antibiotics in patients with total joint replacements is another controversial area. In 2003, the American Dental Association and the American Academy of Orthopaedic Surgeons (AAOS) and their expert panel reviewed the Advisory Statement on Antibiotic Prophylaxis for Dental Patients with Prosthetic Joints originally issued in 1997 and concluded that antibiotic prophylaxis is not indicated for patients with pins, plates, or screws who are undergoing dental extractions, nor is it indicated in those with total joint replacement after 2 years since their implant surgery unless they are in the high-risk category for experiencing hematogenous total joint infection.[17] The latter group included patients with inflammatory arthropathies, drug- or radiation-induced immunosuppression, previous joint infections, malnutrition, hemophilia, HIV infection, insulin-dependent diabetes, or malignancy. However, in 2009, the AAOS issued a statement recommending that clinicians consider antibiotic prophylaxis before performing any invasive procedure that may cause bacteremia in any patient who underwent total joint replacement.[18] This recommendation was made despite the literature supporting the viewpoint that this practice should only be used in high-risk patients.[19,20] Although this is only a recommendation, it raises important medicolegal implications. Based on this, three options have been suggested until this issue is resolved: inform patients about the potential risks involved with antibiotic prophylaxis and let them decide, follow the 2003 guidelines, or suggest to the orthopedic surgeon and patient that they follow the 2003 guidelines.[20]

SUMMARY

Although statements continue to be made in the literature regarding the need for prophylactic antibiotics in certain healthy patients and those with medical risk factors who will be undergoing routine tooth extraction, the studies that have investigated these indications generally seem to indicate that this practice is not actually necessary in most instances. The main indications that seem to be supported by the current literature are for patients with a high risk of endocarditis and those who have had total joint replacements and are at high risk for infection. In the situations that mainly involve opinions expressed in the literature rather than investigative evidence, until controlled studies are performed, practitioners will still have to rely on experience and clinical judgment when making decisions about the use of prophylactic antibiotics.

REFERENCES

1. Epstein JB, Chong S, Le ND. A survey of antibiotic use in dentistry. J Am Dent Assoc 2000;131:1600–9.
2. Alexander RE. Routine prophylactic antibiotic use in diabetic dental patients. J Calif Dent Assoc 1999;8:611–8.
3. Demas PN, McClain JR. Hepatitis: implications for dental care. Oral Surg Oral Med Oral Pathol Oral Radiol Endod 1999;88:2–4.
4. Tong DC, Rothwell BR. Antibiotic prophylaxis in dentistry: a review and practice recommendations. J Am Dent Assoc 2000;131:366–74.
5. Aronovich S, Skope LW, Kelly JP, et al. The relationship of glycemic control to the outcomes of dental extractions. J Oral Maxillofac Surg 2010;68:2955–61.
6. Dodson TB. HIV status and the risk of post-extraction complications. J Dent Res 1977;76:1644–52.
7. Robinson PG, Cooper H, Hatt J. Healing after dental extractions in men with HIV infection. Oral Surg Oral Med Oral Pathol Oral Radiol Endod 1992;74:426–30.
8. Diz Dios P, Feijoo J, Vazquez Garcia E. Tooth extraction in HIV sero-positive patients. Int Dent J 1999;49:317–21.
9. Lockhart PB, Loven B, Brenan MT, et al. The evidence base for the efficacy of antibiotic prophylaxis in dental practice. J Am Dent Assoc 2007;138:48–74.
10. Little JW, Falace DA, Miller CS, et al. Dental management of the medically compromised patient. 7th edition. St Louis (MO): Mosby Inc; 2008.
11. Wilson W, Taubert KA, Gewitz M, et al. Prevention of infective endocarditis: guidelines from the American Heart Association Rheumatic Fever, Endocarditis and Kawasaki Disease Committee, Council on Cardiovascular Disease in the Young, and the Council on Clinical Cardiology, Council on Cardiovascular Surgery and Anesthesia, and the Quality of Care and Outcomes Research Interdisciplinary Working Group. Circulation 2007;116:1736–54.
12. Hong CH, Alfred R, Napenas JJ, et al. Antibiotic prophylaxis for dental procedures to prevent indwelling venous catheter-related infections. Am J Med 2010;123:1128–33.
13. Watson RR, Borgs P, Witte M, et al. Alcohol, immunomodulation, and disease. Alcohol Alcohol 1994;29:131–9.
14. Roda RP, Jimenez Y, Carbonell E, et al. Bacteremia originating in the oral cavity. A review. Med Oral Patol Oral Cir Bucal 2008;13:355–62.
15. Tomas I, Alvarez M, Limeres J, et al. Prevalence, duration and aetiology of bacteremia following dental extractions. Oral Dis 2007;13:56–62.
16. Oliver R, Roberts GJ, Hooper L, et al. Antibiotics for the prophylaxis of bacterial endocarditis in dentistry. Cochrane Database Syst Rev 2008;4:CD003813. DOI:10.1002/14651858.CD003813.pub3.
17. American Dental Association; American Academy of Orthopedic Surgeons. Antibiotic prophylaxis for dental patients with total joint replacements. J Am Dent Assoc 2003;134:805–9.
18. American Academy of Orthopaedic Surgeons Information Statement. Available at: www.aaos.org/about/papers/advistmt/1033.asp. Accessed October 12, 2010.
19. Curry S, Phillips H. Joint arthroplasty, dental treatment, and antibiotics. J Arthroplasty 2002;17:111–3.
20. Little JW, Jacobson JJ, Lockhart PB. The dental treatment of patients with joint replacements: a position paper from the American Academy of Oral Medicine. J Am Dent Assoc 2010;141:667–71.

Do Antibiotics Reduce the Frequency of Surgical Site Infections After Impacted Mandibular Third Molar Surgery?

Srinivas M. Susarla, DMD, MD, MPH[a],*,
Basel Sharaf, DDS, MD[b], Thomas B. Dodson, DMD, MPH[c]

KEYWORDS

- Third molars • Antibiotics • Surgical site infection
- Impacted teeth

The removal of impacted third molars (M3s) represents the cornerstone of oral and maxillofacial ambulatory surgical practice. Although complication rates associated with impacted M3 removal are generally low, the volume of procedures performed is such that small complication rates may affect large absolute numbers of patients. Among the most common complications of impacted M3 removal is postoperative surgical site infection (SSI), with an estimated frequency of 1.2% to 27%, with most studies reporting a frequency of approximately 5%.[1–8] In this setting, significant debate has surrounded the routine use of antibiotics in the management of impacted M3s.[4–6] SSIs can be expensive to manage, especially if hospital admission is required; debilitating to the patient, particularly if further surgery is needed; and, in severe cases, life-threatening if airway compromise or septicemia results. Although these potential issues support the use of antibiotic administration, routine antibiotic treatment, often including broad-spectrum medications, is not without risk. Increasing concerns about the evolution of multidrug-resistant organisms,

adverse reactions to antibiotic use and cost are not trivial. Acknowledging the significant potential risks of antibiotic overuse, the guidelines for endocarditis prophylaxis have been recently revised by the American Heart Association.[9]

The authors address this clinical topic using an evidence-based clinical practice method known as a "critically appraised topic."[10] A critically appraised topic has four components. First, one must translate information needs into an answerable question. Second, one must identify the best available evidence to answer the question. Third, this evidence must be evaluated for its quality (**Table 1**), validity, and applicability. Fourth, the key information must be abstracted, summarized, and transmitted effectively to improve the care of the patients.

MATERIALS AND METHODS

Step 1: Translate Information Needs Into an Answerable Question

This article attempts to answer the following clinical question: "Among patients undergoing the

[a] Department of Oral and Maxillofacial Surgery, Massachusetts General Hospital, 55 Fruit Street, WACC230, Boston, MA 02114, USA
[b] Department of Surgery, School of Medicine and Biomedical Sciences, University at Buffalo, State University of New York, Buffalo General Hospital, 100 High Street, Buffalo, NY 14203, USA
[c] Department of Oral and Maxillofacial Surgery, Center for Applied Clinical Investigation, Massachusetts General Hospital, 55 Fruit Street, Warren 1201, Boston, MA 02114, USA
* Corresponding author.
E-mail address: smsusarla@gmail.com

Oral Maxillofacial Surg Clin N Am 23 (2011) 541–546
doi:10.1016/j.coms.2011.07.007

Table 1 Levels of evidence	
Level of Evidence	**Type of Study**
1a	Systematic reviews of randomized controlled trials
1b	Individual randomized controlled trials
1c	All or none randomized controlled trials
2a	Systematic reviews of cohort studies
2b	Individual cohort study or low quality randomized controlled trials
2c	Outcomes research
3a	Systematic review of case-control studies
3b	Individual case-control study
4	Case series
5	Expert opinion independent of critical appraisal, experimental laboratory research, anecdotal, or "first principles" analyses

Adapted from Oxford Centre for Evidence-Based Medicine, Levels of Evidence. Available at: http://www.cebm.net/index.aspx?o=1025. Accessed March 10, 2011.

removal of impacted mandibular M3s, do those receiving antibiotic therapy, when compared with those who are not, have a decreased risk for SSIs?" In addition, the authors address the issue of method of antibiotic administration (systemic vs topical) and timing of administration. The types of antibiotics typically used are not discussed, because this topic is addressed elsewhere in this issue. This article focuses on impacted mandibular third molars, because most infections associated with impacted tooth removal occur in these teeth.[1,2] Finally, the effectiveness of antibiotic prophylaxis on the frequency of SSIs after erupted M3 removal is not addressed, because it has been well-established that SSIs are associated with impacted M3s.[1,2] Finally, SSIs are only addressed, not alveolar osteitis.

Step 2: Identify the Best Evidence to Answer the Question

To identify the best evidence to answer the aforementioned clinical question, the authors conducted a computerized literature search of Medline (using Ovid as the search engine), PubMed, and the Cochrane Central Register of Controlled Trials

with a combination of Medical Subject Headings, including "antibiotics," "antibacterial agents," "antimicrobial agents," and "third molars." The authors evaluated the abstracts from the query results and selected articles that were described as a randomized controlled clinical trial (RCT) or a review with meta-analyses of the same, and included SSI as an outcome. Studies that did not involve a control group, had no randomization of subjects to intervention and control arms, and did not define the outcome were not included.

Step 3: Appraise the Literature

This search identified 114 studies. The studies selected for inclusion in this review included one review with a meta-analysis of 12 RCTs (**Table 2**).[4,7,8,11–21] One RCT included in the meta-analysis as an abstract was subsequently published in a peer-reviewed journal.[16] Another RCT was identified that was published after the meta-analysis.[22] Two RCTs using topical antibiotics were identified but excluded because the primary outcome was alveolar osteitis.[23,24]

RESULTS
Step 4: Abstract the Key Information, Summarize the Information, and Transmit the Information to Improve the Care of the Patients

Data pertaining to the 12 RCTs evaluating the efficacy of systemic antibiotic therapy in the removal of impacted third molars are summarized in **Table 1**. Among the 12 RCTs, 2396 subjects were randomized to receive systemic antibiotics (n = 1110) or to a control group (n = 1286). Within the treatment group, wound infections occurred in 44 subjects (4.0%) receiving systemic antibiotics and 78 subjects (6.1%) receiving no antibiotic therapy. The use of systemic antibiotics had a 35% lower risk of postoperative SSI (relative risk, 0.65; 95% CI, 0.46, 0.94).

Ren and Malmstrom[11] meta-analyzed these 12 clinical trials in 2007 and found no significant heterogeneity among the studies ($P = .26$), suggesting that the results could be pooled. In addition, the publication bias assessment score was relatively low (13), suggesting a low probability of publication bias. They found that, to prevent one case of postoperative SSI, 25 patients would require systemic antibiotics (ie, the number needed to treat was 25).

Since the publication of this meta-analysis, one RCT evaluating systemic antibiotic prophylaxis in M3 surgery has been published.[22] Using a split-mouth design, Siddiqi and colleagues[22] conducted a clinical trial of 100 healthy subjects. Each

Table 2
Summary of randomized controlled clinical trials evaluating prophylactic antibiotic efficacy in impacted mandibular third molar surgery

Author	Study Groups	Route	Timing	No. of Subjects	No. of Infections	ARR[a]	NNT[b]
Mitchell,[19] 1986	Tinidazole, 2000 mg[c]	po	Pre	25	0	0.16	6
	Placebo			25	4		
Lombardia Garcia et al,[20] 1987	Amoxicillin, 500 mg	po	Pre	44	1	<0.01	500
	No intervention			441	11		
Graziani et al,[15] 2005	Azithromycin, 500 mg × 3 d	po	Pre	20	0	0.10	10
	Control			10	1		
Halpern and Dodson,[8] 2007	Penicillin, 15 KU/kg[d]	IV	Pre	59	0	0.09	11
	Placebo			59	5		
Lacasa et al,[16] 2003, 2007	Augmentin, 2000/125 mg	po	Pre	75	4	0.11	9
	Augmentin, 2000/125 mg × 5 d	po	Post	75	2	0.13	8
	Placebo			75	12		
Monaco et al,[13] 1999	Amoxicillin, 2000 mg × 5 d	po	Post	66	2	0.08	13
	No intervention			75	8		
Poeschl et al,[4] 2004	Augmentin, 500/125 mg × 5 d	po	Post	176	6	0.01	143
	Clindamycin, 300 mg × 5 d	po	Post	180	8	0.00	e
	No intervention			172	7		
Arteagoitia et al,[14] 2005	Augmentin, 500/125 mg × 4 d	po	Post	231	5	0.02	50
	Placebo			259	11		
Curran et al,[7] 1974	Penicillin G, 1 million IU + 250 mg × 4 d	IM/po	Pre + Post	33	0	0.09	12
	No intervention			35	3		
Bystedt et al,[21] 1980	Azidocillin,750 mg + erythromycin, 500/250 mg Clindamycin, 300/150 mg, and doxycycline, 200/100 mg × 7 d	po	Pre + Post	80	2	0.11	9
	Placebo			60	8		
Happonen et al,[12] 1990	Pen VK, 660 mg × 5 d	po	Pre + Post	44	6	−0.03	e
	Tinidazole, 500 mg × 5 d[c]	po	Pre + Post	47	5	0.01	200
	Placebo			45	5		
Bulut et al,[18] 2001	Amoxicillin, 500 mg × 4 d	po	Pre + Post	30	2	0.00	f
	Placebo			30	2		

Abbreviations: ARR, absolute risk reduction; IM, intramuscularly; IV, intravenously; NNT, number needed to treat; Pen VK, penicillin V potassium; Pre, preoperatively; Post, postoperatively.
  [a] ARR: difference between the risk of infection with no intervention/placebo versus antibiotic.
  [b] NNT: number of patients who would require antibiotic treatment to prevent one SSI.
  [c] Regimen not currently available.
  [d] For patients allergic to penicillin, 600 mg of clindamycin was administered.
  [e] ARR suggests detrimental use of antibiotic (ie, rate of SSI higher in antibiotic group). For all ARR in this group, *P*>.05.
  [f] NNT not calculated for risk difference of zero.

participant underwent unilateral extraction of impacted M3s during the first surgical visit, with subsequent extraction of the contralateral impacted M3s 3 weeks later. Subjects were randomized into two study groups. In the first, systemic antibiotics were given as a single dose preoperatively on either the first or second visit, with placebo given when antibiotic was not. In the second group, a systemic antibiotic was administered preoperatively and for 2 days postoperatively at the first surgical visit. No antibiotic was given at the second surgical visit. All impacted M3s were removed using a standard surgical technique under local anesthesia. Among subjects who received preoperative antibiotics only, four postoperative infections occurred, three of which occurred during the placebo phase. Among subjects who received perioperative antibiotics on the first visit and placebo on the second visit, one infection occurred on the third day after surgery with perioperative antibiotics. These authors found an overall infection rate of 2%, with no significant difference noted between antibiotic and placebo ($P>.05$).

The results of this small trial could not be pooled with the data from the prior meta-analysis because whether the infections occurred in mandibular or maxillary surgical sites was unknown. However, the low infection rate in the setting of a small sample of patients suggests that sample-size effects could influence the results in this trial. In addition, the study design, which involved a split-mouth technique under local anesthesia, although adequate for epidemiologic purposes, limits the generalizability of this study with regard to the population of patients undergoing M3 extraction in the United States.

Timing of Antibiotics

Of the RCTs evaluated herein, multiple dosing strategies were used for antibiotic use (see **Table 1**): single-dose preoperative administration, multidose preoperative administration, perioperative dosing (preoperative and postoperative continuous dosing), and multiday postoperative dosing only. Among the RCTs included in the meta-analysis, systemic antibiotics were shown to be effective in preventing SSI only when started preoperatively and continued postoperatively. The meta-analysis concluded that single-dose preoperative administrations, multidose preoperative administrations, and postoperative administrations were not effective. However, a well-designed and implemented RCT, representative of ambulatory oral surgery practice in the United States, showed a reduction in SSIs using a single dose of intravenous penicillin (or clindamycin) preoperatively.[8]

Route of Antibiotic Administration

Among the well-designed and implemented clinical trials to date, varying antibiotic routes have been used. Most use oral antibiotics, but two RCTs identified used intramuscular or intravenous antibiotics. In the first, a single dose of intramuscular penicillin was administered preoperatively, followed by a 4-day course of oral penicillin.[7] The results of this trial did not show a significant difference in infection rates (0% vs 8.7%; $P = .23$). However, this was a relatively small trial, with 33 subjects receiving intervention and 35 subjects receiving placebo. A second trial studied the effectiveness of a single dose of intravenous penicillin administered 30 minutes preoperatively.[8] No postoperative antibiotics were given. This study showed a higher rate of SSI in the placebo group (8.5% vs 0%; $P = .03$). This well-designed and well-conducted trial concluded that a single intravenous dose of penicillin resulted in a lower rate of postoperative SSI.

DISCUSSION

Despite 60 years of clinical experience with systemic antibiotics, and numerous well-designed and implemented clinical studies, significant debate remains over the indications for prophylactic antibiotics in impacted mandibular M3 surgery. The controversy has continued for several reasons. First, although many studies addressing this question have had good-to-excellent internal validity, external validity has been a significant problem. Specifically, many completed studies were conducted in settings that are significantly dissimilar to those of contemporary American oral surgical practice. These studies have been completed on subjects who have M3s extracted under local anesthesia or in a dedicated operating room under general anesthesia (60% of patients receive intravenous sedation for these procedures in the United States), either one at a time or as unilateral extractions (multiple M3s are usually extracted in a single-visit). Second, many trials have used antibiotic regimens and dosing strategies and intervals that are generally nonstandard. The effectiveness of prophylactic antibiotics relies on administration before incision, so that adequate systemic concentrations are achieved before inoculation of the wound and bloodstream with microorganisms. The most commonly used antibiotics to prevent postoperative SSIs are penicillin and clindamycin. Several trials have either used different antibiotics or nonstandard regimens (eg, postoperative dosing only). Independent of these characteristics, a well-done meta-analysis has shown a significant benefit to antibiotic use in preventing SSI after extraction of impacted mandibular M3s.

With regard to risk/benefit analyses, available data from well-designed RCTs suggest that 10 to 25 individuals would require antibiotic treatment to prevent one SSI. The estimated incidence of common side effects (eg, diarrhea, nausea, rashes, vomiting, vaginitis) with amoxicillin/clindamycin is approximately 1% to 3% (ie, of 100 patients treated with prophylactic doses of such antibiotics, 1–3 would experience a side effect).[25–27] In this setting, the use of prophylactic antibiotics is justified as having a greater benefit than potential harm.

What is the practitioner to make of these perplexing and conflicting data? Using the best available data pertaining to practice patterns in the United States, which include multiple M3s extracted in a single setting under ambulatory anesthesia (ie, intravenous sedation), level I evidence suggests patients will benefit from a single dose of systemic antibiotic administered preoperatively.[8] Therefore, the authors recommend that for otherwise healthy patients undergoing extraction of at least one impacted mandibular M3 in the ambulatory setting, a single-dose of intravenous penicillin or clindamycin be used to prevent postoperative SSI. Oral systemic antibiotic therapy should be administered preoperatively and continued postoperatively for 2 to 7 days. For patients undergoing M3 extraction in settings that deviate significantly from this, good-quality data are insufficient to make specific recommendations. Future studies are needed to evaluate the efficacy of antibiotic use in other settings, including topical antibiotics and the use of antibiotics in patients with preexisting infections and pericoronitis.

REFERENCES

1. Susarla SM, Blaeser BF, Magalnick D. Third molar surgery and associated complications. Oral Maxillofac Surg Clin North Am 2003;15(2):177–86.
2. Chuang SK, Perrott DH, Susarla SM, et al. Risk factors for inflammatory complications following third molar surgery in adults. J Oral Maxillofac Surg 2008;66(11):2213–8.
3. Lieblich SE. Postoperative prophylactic antibiotic treatment in third molar surgery—a necessity? J Oral Maxillofac Surg 2004;62:9.
4. Poeschl PW, Eckel D, Poeschl E. Postoperative prophylactic antibiotic treatment in third molar surgery—a necessity? J Oral Maxillofac Surg 2004;62:3–8.
5. Piecuch JF, Arzadon J, Lieblich SE. Prophylactic antibiotics for third molar surgery: a supporting opinion. J Oral Maxillofac Surg 1995;53:53.
6. Zeitler DL. Prophylactic antibiotics for third molar surgery: a dissenting opinion. J Oral Maxillofac Surg 1995;53:61.
7. Curran JB, Kennett S, Young AR. An assessment of the use of prophylactic antibiotics in third molar surgery. Int J Oral Surg 1974;3:1.
8. Halpern LR, Dodson TB. Does prophylactic administration of systemic antibiotics prevent postoperative inflammatory complications after third molar surgery? J Oral Maxillofac Surg 2007;65:177.
9. Wilson W, Taubert KA, Gewitz M, et al. Prevention of infective endocarditis: guidelines from the American Heart Association: a guideline from the American Heart Association Rheumatic Fever, Endocarditis and Kawasaki Disease Committee, Council on Cardiovascular Disease in the Young, and the Council on Clinical Cardiology, Council on Cardiovascular Surgery and Anesthesia, and the Quality of Care and Outcomes Research Interdisciplinary Working Group. J Am Dent Assoc 2007;138(6): 739–45, 747–60.
10. Dodson TB, Richardson DT. Risk of periodontal defects after third molar surgery: an exercise in evidence-based clinical decision-making. Oral Maxillofac Surg Clin North Am 2007;19(1):93–8, vii.
11. Ren YF, Malmstrom HS. Effectiveness of antibiotic prophylaxis in third molar surgery: a meta-analysis of randomized controlled clinical trials. J Oral Maxillofac Surg 2007;65(10):1909–21.
12. Happonen RP, Backstrom AC, Ylipaavalniemi P. Prophylactic use of phenoxymethylpenicillin and tinidazole in mandibular third molar surgery, a comparative placebo controlled clinical trial. Br J Oral Maxillofac Surg 1990;28:12.
13. Monaco G, Staffolani C, Gatto MR, et al. Antibiotic therapy in impacted third molar surgery. Eur J Oral Sci 1999;107:437.
14. Arteagoitia I, Diez A, Barbier L, et al. Efficacy of amoxicillin/clavulanic acid in preventing infectious and inflammatory complications following impacted mandibular third molar extraction. Oral Surg Oral Med Oral Pathol Oral Radiol Endod 2005;100:e11.
15. Graziani F, Corsi L, Fornai M, et al. Clinical evaluation of piroxicam-FDDF and azithromycin in the prevention of complications associated with impacted lower third molar extraction. Pharmacol Res 2005;52:485.
16. Lacasa JM, Jiménez JA, Ferrás V, et al. Prophylaxis versus pre-emptive treatment for infective and inflammatory complications of surgical third molar removal: a randomized, double-blind, placebo-controlled, clinical trial with sustained release amoxicillin/clavulanic acid (1000/62.5 mg). Int J Oral Maxillofac Surg 2007;36(4):321–7.
17. Bergdahl M, Hedstrom L. Metronidazole for the prevention of dry socket after removal of partially impacted mandibular third molar: a randomized

controlled trial. Br J Oral Maxillofac Surg 2004; 42:555.

18. Bulut E, Bulut S, Etikan I, et al. The value of routine antibiotic prophylaxis in mandibular third molar surgery: acute-phase protein levels as indicators of infection. J Oral Sci 2001;43:117.

19. Mitchell DA. A controlled clinical trial of prophylactic tinidazole for chemoprophylaxis in third molar surgery. Br Dent J 1986;160:284.

20. Lombardia Garcia E, Garcia Pola MJ, Gonzalez Garcia M, et al. Antimicrobial prophylaxis in surgery of the third molar. Analytic study of post-operative complications. Arch Odonto Estomatol 1987;3:130 [in Spanish].

21. Bystedt H, Nord CE, Nordenram A. Effect of azido-cillin, erythromycin, clindamycin and doxycycline on postoperative complications after surgical removal of impacted mandibular third molars. Int J Oral Surg 1980;9:157.

22. Siddiqi A, Morkel JA, Zafar S. Antibiotic prophylaxis in third molar surgery: a randomized double-blind placebo-controlled clinical trial using split-mouth technique. Int J Oral Maxillofac Surg 2010;39(2): 107–14.

23. Schatz JP, Fiore-Donno G, Henning G. Fibrinolytic alveolitis and its prevention. Int J Oral Maxillofac Surg 1987;16:175.

24. MacGregor AJ, Hutchinson D. The effect of sulfon-amides on pain and swelling following removal of ectopic third molars. Int J Oral Surg 1975;4:184.

25. Salvo F, De Sarro A, Caputi AP, et al. Amoxicillin and amoxicillin plus clavulanate: a safety review. Expert Opin Drug Saf 2009;8(1):111–8.

26. Walker CB. Selected antimicrobial agents: mecha-nisms of action, side effects and drug interactions. Periodontol 2000 1996;10:12–28.

27. Kasten MJ. Clindamycin, metronidazole, and chlor-amphenicol. Mayo Clin Proc 1999;74:825–33.

Does the Use of Prophylactic Antibiotics Decrease Implant Failure?

Basel Sharaf, DDS, MD[a],*, Thomas B. Dodson, DMD, MPH[b]

KEYWORDS

- Prophylactic antibiotics • Implant dentistry • Implant failure
- Dental implants

The use of dental implants in oral rehabilitation is widely accepted, with an estimated 1 million dental implants placed annually worldwide.[1–5] Despite a high success rate, implant failures do occur. Failure of dental implants can be attributable to implant-related, patient-related, and surgical technique–related factors.[5] Bacterial colonization of the implant surface and surgical site infection have been implicated in early implant failure.[6] Once an infection ensues at the implant site, eradication of the infection is usually difficult, which may lead to the ultimate removal of the implant.[6] For this reason, various antibiotic regimens, including multiday perioperative regimens to a single preoperative dose have been suggested to minimize early infections after dental implant placement. However, the routine use of antibiotics is not without risks. Complications including gastrointestinal symptoms to more serious allergic reactions are not uncommon. In addition, the selection of antibiotic-resistant bacteria is a major public health concern. The purpose of this article is to answer the following question: "In patients receiving dental implants, does the administration of prophylactic antibiotics reduce early implant failure?"

MATERIAL AND METHODS

To answer the question, the authors searched the Medline English language literature with PubMed and the Cochrane Central Register of Controlled Trials (CENTRAL). The authors searched using the following Medical Subject Headings (MeSH): antimicrobial agents, antibiotics or prophylactic antibiotics, and dental implants. All relevant studies published in English through December 2010 were included. Fifty-nine articles met the initial screening criteria. Abstracts from the search query were reviewed. Articles meeting the following criteria were selected: (1) randomized controlled clinical trials, (2) meta-analysis or systematic review. The primary predictor variable was antibiotic therapy, classified as a preoperative dose of antibiotics, preoperative and postoperative antibiotic treatment, and no antibiotics. The primary outcome variable was implant failure. The secondary outcome variable was postoperative infection. Each article was reviewed and data summarized for the following variables: sample size, antibiotic use, implant failure, and postoperative infections. The treatment effect was measured using absolute risk reduction (ARR), which is defined

[a] Department of Surgery, School of Medicine and Biomedical Sciences, University at Buffalo, State University of New York, Buffalo General Hospital, Buffalo, NY, USA
[b] Department of Oral and Maxillofacial Surgery, Center for Applied Clinical Investigation, Harvard School of Dental Medicine and Massachusetts General Hospital, Warren Building-Suite 1201, 55 Fruit Street, Boston, MA 02114, USA
* Corresponding author. Department of Surgery, Buffalo General Hospital, 100 High Street Room C381, Buffalo, NY 14203.
E-mail address: sharafddsmd@gmail.com

Oral Maxillofacial Surg Clin N Am 23 (2011) 547–550
doi:10.1016/j.coms.2011.07.008

as the absolute difference in failure rates between the intervention and control groups. The number needed to treat (NNT), calculated as the reciprocal of ARR, is defined as the number of implants that must be placed with antibiotic use to prevent 1 implant failure.

RESULTS

Five articles were selected for review.[7–11] Four studies were randomized controlled trials (RCTs, level of evidence 1b),[12] and are summarized in **Table 1**. One study was a meta-analysis (Cochrane systematic review) of these 4 RCTs (level of evidence 1a).[11]

The first RCT, by Abu Ta'a and colleagues,[7] compared 1 g of amoxicillin given 1 hour preoperatively and 500 mg of amoxicillin 4 times daily given for 2 days postoperatively versus no antibiotics. All patients rinsed with chlorhexidine once before implant placement and twice daily for 7 to 10 days postoperatively. Each group included 40 patients and there were a total of 247 implants inserted. At 5 months follow-up, 5 implants failed in 3 patients who did not receive antibiotics (5 of 119 implants failed; ARR 4.2%). There were no failures in the antibiotic group. Four patients in the untreated group and 1 patient in the antibiotic group developed postoperative infection. The differences were not statistically significant between the 2 groups for any of the outcome measures.

Esposito and colleagues,[8,9] in 2 consecutive RCTs, compared the effect of 2 g of amoxicillin given 1 hour preoperatively with placebo tablets. All patients received oral hygiene instructions and professional dental debridement 1 week before implant insertion. In addition, all patients rinsed with chlorhexidine preoperatively and twice daily for 7 days postoperatively. In the first study,[8] 165 patients were included in each group with a total of 696 implants placed. There were 9 implant failures in the control group and 2 implant failures in the antibiotic group (ARR 1.9%). Three patients in the antibiotic group developed infection versus 2 patients in the placebo group. In the second study,[9] 252 patients were included in the antibiotic group and 254 patients in the control group, with a total of 972 implants placed. Five patients in the antibiotic group experienced 7 implant failures, whereas 12 patients in the placebo group had 13 implant failures (ARR 1.3%). In both studies, there were no statistically significant differences for implant failure or postoperative infection between the 2 groups.

Anitua and colleagues[10] compared 2 g of amoxicillin given 1 hour preoperatively with placebo tablets. All patients received oral hygiene instructions and dental prophylaxis a few days before implant placement. Patients rinsed with chlorhexidine before surgery. Only single implants placed in medium-quality bone were included. In addition, implants were treated with autologous plasma rich in growth factors. Fifty-two patients were included in the antibiotic group and 53 patients in the control group. Two patients in each group lost their implants and 6 patients in each group had postoperative infections. There were no statistically significant differences in outcome measured between the 2 groups.

A meta-analysis of the 4 RCTs included 1007 patients and a total of 2020 implants.[11] There were more implant failures in the control group (not receiving antibiotics), with a statistically significant difference between the 2 groups after pooling the patient groups from the 4 RCTs (risk ratio 0.40, 95% confidence interval [CI] 0.19–0.84). The number of patients needed to be treated with antibiotics to prevent 1 patient from having implant failure was 33 (95% CI 17–100).[11] There were no statistically significant differences for the other outcomes, including prosthesis failure, postoperative infection, and adverse events.

DISCUSSION

The purpose of this study was to answer the question: Does antibiotic therapy, when given either as a single dose preoperatively or multiday treatment postoperatively, decrease the failure rate of dental implants? To answer this question, the authors used a comprehensive literature review. Three of the 4 individual RCTs showed a trend toward reduction of implant failure when antibiotics were used, although the differences between the groups were not statistically significant. This is consistent with our findings in a previous literature review.[13] One RCT included patients with medium-quality bone in whom a single implant was placed in conjunction with plasma rich in growth factors. This study failed to show a difference between the 2 groups. When the 4 RCTs were combined in a meta-analysis, however, a statistically significant reduction in implant failure was observed when patients received 2 g of amoxicillin 1 hour preoperatively or 1 g of amoxicillin administered 1 hour preoperatively and 500 mg 4 times daily for 2 days postoperatively. The number of patients needed to be treated with antibiotics to prevent 1 patient from early implant loss was 33. There were no major adverse effects related to antibiotic use reported in the 4 RCTs. There is paucity of evidence to support the routine use of postoperative antibiotics. This is reflected by 2 prospective studies comparing the effect of preoperative antibiotics versus postoperative antibiotics only.[1,4]

Table 1
Summary of randomized controlled trials

Study	Follow-up Period (months)	Sample Size (Implants, Patients)	No Ab % Failure[a]	Preop Ab % Failure	Preop & Postop Ab % Failure	ARR	NNT
Abu-Ta'a et al,[7] 2008	5	247 (implants) / 80 (patients)	4.2% (5/119 implants) / 7.5% (3/40 patients)	N/A[b]	0% (0/128 implants) / 0% (0/40 patients)	4.2% (implants) / 7.5% (patients)	24 (implants) / 13 (patients)
Esposito et al,[8] 2008	4	696 (implants) / 316 (patients)	2.5% (9/355 implants) / 5.1% (8/158 patients)	0.6% (2/341 implants) / 1.3% (2/159 patients)	N/A	1.9% (implants) / 3.8% (patients)	52 (implants) / 27 (patients)
Anitua et al,[10] 2009	3	105 (implants) / 105 (patients)	3.8% (2/53 implants)	3.8% (2/52 implants)	N/A	N/A	N/A
Esposito et al,[9] 2010	4	972 (implants) / 506 (patients)	2.7% (13/483 implants) / 4.7% (12/254 patients)	1.4% (7/489 implants) / 2% (5/252 patients)	N/A	1.3% (implants) / 2.7% (patients)	76 (implants) / 37 (patients)

Abbreviations: Ab, Antibiotics; ARR, absolute risk reduction; NNT, number of implants needed to be placed in conjunction with antibiotics to prevent 1 implant failure.
[a] Percentage failure is the number of failed implants divided by total implants in the group.
[b] Not applicable.

Dent and colleagues[1] demonstrated that when preoperative antibiotics were used, there was 1.5% implant failure compared with a 4.0% failure rate when only postoperative antibiotics were used in an 800-patient study. Laskin and colleagues[4] reported higher failure rates (10%) when only postoperative antibiotics were given compared with preoperative antibiotics (4.6%).

There are some drawbacks to the RCTs reviewed. The follow-up time varied from 3 months in 1 trial[10] and 4 months in 2 trials[4,9] to 5 months in 1 trial.[3] Decreasing the follow-up period may decrease the number of failed implants and may overestimate the effect of antibiotics on the primary outcome variable: implant failure. Another drawback is the use of bone substitutes and other bone-regenerative procedures at the time of implant placement, which may affect implant healing and failure rates. The use of bone-regenerative procedures was reported in 2 studies.[7,10] In addition, the effect of timing of implant placement (delayed or immediately after extraction) may potentially increase implant failure rates. Esposito and colleagues[9] demonstrated in a logistic regression analysis that patients in the RCT who received immediate postextraction implants had a 9% failure rate versus 2% in the delayed group, regardless of antibiotic use ($P<.001$).[9]

SUMMARY

Based on the 4 reviewed RCTs and the meta-analysis, there is evidence that the use of a single preoperative dose of 2 g amoxicillin 1 hour before implant placement or 1 g amoxicillin 1 hour preoperatively and 500 mg 4 times daily for 2 days postoperatively can significantly reduce the rate of early implant failure. To prevent 1 patient from implant failure, 33 patients must be treated with antibiotics. The use of antibiotics has no statistically significant effect on postoperative infections after implant placement. Based on these findings, the authors recommend the following: in otherwise healthy patients who are not allergic to penicillin, a 2 g preoperative dose of amoxicillin, or a 1 g preoperative dose of amoxicillin and 500 mg 4 times daily for 2 days postoperatively is recommended to prevent early implant failure. In clinical settings that diverge from that scenario, the clinician's own judgment of each individual patient is essential in tailoring antibiotic use to prevent implant infection and failure.

A large double-blind, randomized controlled trial comparing the use of a standardized antibiotic regimen (preoperative and/or postoperative) versus placebo is needed to further elucidate the most efficacious antibiotic regimen in reducing early dental implant failure.[13]

REFERENCES

1. Dent CD, Olson JW, Farish SE, et al. The influence of preoperative antibiotics on success of endosseous implants up to and including stage II surgery: a study of 2,641 implants. J Oral Maxillofac Surg 1997;55(12 Suppl 5):19–24.
2. Gynther GW, Köndell PA, Moberg LE, et al. Dental implant installation without antibiotic prophylaxis. Oral Surg Oral Med Oral Pathol Oral Radiol Endod 1998;85(5):509–11.
3. Binahmed A, Stoykewych A, Peterson L. Single preoperative dose versus long-term prophylactic antibiotic regimens in dental implant surgery. Int J Oral Maxillofac Implants 2005;20(1):115–7.
4. Laskin DM, Dent CD, Morris HF, et al. The influence of preoperative antibiotics on success of endosseous implants at 36 months. Ann Periodontol 2000;5(1):166–74.
5. Pye AD, Lockhart DE, Dawson MP, et al. A review of dental implants and infection. J Hosp Infect 2009; 72:104–10.
6. Esposito M, Hirsch JM, Lekholm U, et al. Biological factors contributing to failures of osseointegrated oral implants. (II) Etiopathogenesis. Eur J Oral Sci 1998;106:721–64.
7. Abu-Ta'a M, Quirynen M, Teughels W, et al. Asepsis during periodontal surgery involving oral implants and the usefulness of peri-operative antibiotics: a prospective, randomized, controlled clinical trial. J Clin Periodontol 2008;35(1):58–63.
8. Esposito M, Cannizzaro G, Bozzoli P, et al. Efficacy of prophylactic antibiotics for dental implants: a multicentre placebo-controlled randomised clinical trial. Eur J Oral Implantol 2008;1:23–31.
9. Esposito M, Cannizzaro G, Bozzoli P, et al. Effectiveness of prophylactic antibiotics at placement of dental implants: a pragmatic multicenter placebo-controlled randomized clinical trial. Eur J Oral Implantol 2010;3(2):135–43.
10. Anitua E, Aguirre JJ, Gorosable A, et al. A multicenter placebo-controlled randomized clinical trial of antibiotic prophylaxis for placement of single dental implants. Eur J Oral Implantol 2009;2:283–92.
11. Esposito M, Worthington HV, Loli V, et al. Interventions for replacing missing teeth: antibiotics at dental implant placement to prevent complications (Review). Cochrane Database Syst Rev 2010;7:CD004152.
12. Center of Evidence Based Medicine. Available at: http://www.cebm.net/levels_of_evidence. Accessed January 27, 2011.
13. Sharaf B, Jandali Rifai M, Dodson TB. Do perioperative antibiotics decrease implant failure? J Oral Maxillofac Surg 2011;69(9):2345–50.

How Can We As Dentists Minimize Our Contribution to the Problem of Antibiotic Resistance?

Drew B. Havard, DMD, J. Michael Ray, DDS*

KEYWORDS

- Antibiotic resistance • Odontogenic infection • Biofilms

The discovery of antibiotics in the early 20th century was not only a turning point in medicine, but in human history as well. A serious consequence of the use of these lifesaving and wondrous medicines, appropriate or otherwise, has been the development of resistance. Bacterial resistance to antibiotics is multifactorial. In medicine, antibiotic resistance has been attributed to long-term and repetitive use of broad-spectrum antibiotics.[1] Some resistance occurs intrinsically, but much of the blame is attributable to decades of use by medical practitioners, nontherapeutic use in agriculture, and careless disposal of waste by the pharmaceutical industry as a whole.

The first discovered antimicrobial family, the sulfonamides, were reported and became available for commercial use in 1937. Penicillin became mass-produced in the 1940s and available to the American public in the 1950s without a prescription and was widely used to treat a wide array of infections and other maladies. But only a few years after the discovery of antibiotics, resistance to these drugs and their mechanism of resistance were reported. Mutant strains of *Mycobacterium tuberculosis* were identified shortly after streptomycin was introduced in 1944 that were resistant to the therapeutic levels used to treat tuberculosis.[2] Over the next several decades, the discovery of new antimicrobial agents was soon followed by the discovery of resistant organisms. This problem has proved to be unrelenting and a constant source of frustration for researchers, health care providers, and patients alike.

Ingestion of food animals treated with prophylactic or therapeutic dosings of antibiotics may add to the problem of antibiotic exposure and eventual resistance in humans. Although the agriculture and animal husbandry industry uses massive amounts of antibiotics, the actual quantity is difficult to assess and compare. The most recent data reported by the Food and Drug Administration (FDA) on the quantity of antibiotics sold and distributed in the United States for food production are listed in **Table 1**. The FDA estimates that more than 13 million kilograms of antibiotics (nearly 29 million pounds) were sold and distributed for animal use in food production.[3] In comparison of these data with a recent estimate of antibiotic use in humans of approximately 3 million pounds annually in the United States, one can loosely extrapolate that the agricultural industry may use upwards of 90% of all antibiotics distributed in the United States.[4] The relative proportion of antibiotic use in humans and animals is illustrated in **Fig. 1**. The use of antibiotics in such massive quantities has undoubtedly contributed to resistant bacteria in chickens, swine, and cattle, but the impact of this on humans has been difficult

The authors have nothing to disclose.
Department of Oral and Maxillofacial Surgery, Baylor College of Dentistry, Texas A&M Health Science Center, 3302 Gaston Avenue, Dallas, TX 75246, USA
* Corresponding author.
E-mail address: mray@bcd.tamhsc.edu

oralmaxsurgery.theclinics.com

Table 1
Antimicrobial drugs approved for domestic use in food-producing animals: 2009 sales and distribution data reported by drug class from the Food and Drug Administration summary report on antimicrobials sold or distributed for use in food-producing animals

Antimicrobial Class	Annual Totals, kg
Aminoglycosides	339,678
Cephalosporins	41,328
Ionophores	3,740,627
Licosamides	115,837
Macrolides	861,985
Penicillins	610,514
Sulfas	517,873
Tetracyclines	4,611,892
NIR[a]	2,227,366

[a] NIR, not independently reported. Antimicrobial classes for which there were less than 3 distinct sponsors actively marketing products domestically were not independently reported. These classes include Aminocoumarins, Amphenicols, Diaminopyrimidines, Fluroquinolones, Glycolipids, Pleuromutilins, Polypeptides, Quinoxalines, and Streptogramins.

to directly ascertain.[5] Food poisoning caused by fluoroquinolone-resistant *Campylobacter. jejuni* has been reported and extensively analyzed. The FDA has reported that about 8000 to 10,000 persons per year are infected by fluoroquinolone-resistant *C jejuni* from chicken.[6] Even more disturbing is that the same resistant strains responsible for infections in humans were found in the raw meat of chicken.[7] Even when food animals are not therapeutically treated with antibiotics for infections, antibiotics enter the food environment through the animals' food and water sources, thus providing another means of passing antibiotics and potentially resistant bacteria to humans.[8] The extensive use of nontherapeutic (prophylactic) antibiotics in animal agriculture in food animals, to compensate for infections related to unsanitary conditions and to synthetic feeds designed to accelerate muscle growth, causes contamination of environmental water supplies and the entire food chain. This "cycle" of contamination of the environment with trace antibiotics and resistant bacteria is illustrated in **Fig. 2**.

It is difficult to estimate the amount of antibiotic compounds released into the environment in the form of manufacturing waste products, but the quantity is likely in the many millions of metric tons.[2] Many of these noxious compounds are resistant to biodegradation and therefore accumulate in soil, rivers, and reservoirs. One of the most shocking examples of this are the results from water samples taken near a major pharmaceutical manufacturing plant in Hyderabad, India, in 2009.[9] Lakes nearby not known to be contaminated by the plant's effluent demonstrated concentrations

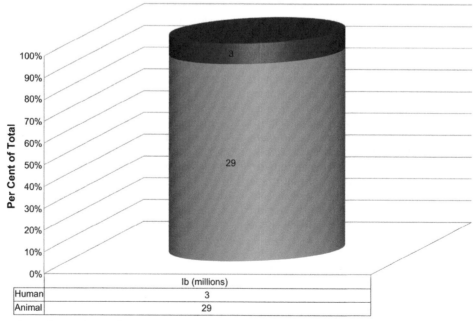

Fig. 1. Estimated annual use of antibiotics per year in the United States, in millions of pounds, for human therapeutic purposes (9% of total) versus animal feed supplements (91% of total). (*Courtesy of* Thomas R. Flynn, DMD.)

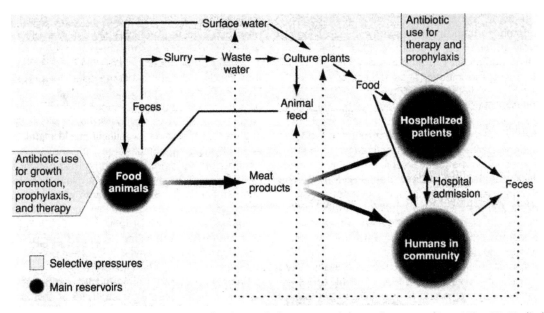

Fig. 2. Interaction of antibiotics, bacteria, food animals, humans, and the environment. (*From* Witte W. Medical consequences of antibiotic use in agriculture. Science 1998;279:996–7; with permission.)

of ciprofloxacin of up to 6.5 mg/L. This alarmingly high concentration suggests the plant's effluent alone is not responsible for such contamination and that other sources are contributing. Although this may seem an extreme example, similar stories are probably untold throughout the world.

Antibiotic resistance occurs by both intrinsic defenses and by genetic mutation in bacteria. The mutations happen both spontaneously and as a result of horizontal gene transfer. Planktonic bacteria typically acquire resistance in 1 of 4 ways: (1) alteration of a drug's target site, (2) inability of a drug to reach target site, (3) inactivation of an antimicrobial agent, or (4) active elimination of an antibiotic from the cell. Gene transfer via plasmids results in a change of the microbe's DNA, and the resistant genes are passed to subsequent generations.

It is important to understand that infections of the oral cavity are not caused by planktonic, or "free-floating," bacteria. Rather, all infections encountered in the practice of dentistry are caused by bacteria that live and flourish in a biofilm. A biofilm is a highly organized community of a multitude of bacterial species that are surrounded and protected by an exopolysaccharide produced by the resident bacteria. Bacteria that began as free-floating bacteria come in contact with a surface and become adherent. Immediately, these newly attached bacteria begin laying down an exopolymeric matrix that provides additional surface area for the attachment of other bacteria

and provide a means of trapping nutrients. Within the biofilm lie water channels that allow for the flow of nutrients and for the elimination of waste products.

Bacteria in a biofilm are uniquely resistant to conventional antibiotics even beyond the mechanisms of antibiotic resistance discussed previously. Bacteria communicate with each other via numerous complex mechanisms, including quorum sensing, a complex method of alteration of gene expression and gene transfer even among different species of bacteria and nanowiring involving electrically conductive pili used for long-range electrical and energy transfer. The exopolysaccharide may also provide a resistant barrier to some antibiotics.

The spread of biofilm bacteria occurs by 3 means: expansion of bacteria within the biofilm, detachment of bacterial "clumps," or shear from environmental flow forces. Even as the bacteria may once again become planktonic before they reattach, they retain the biofilm-specific resistance genes and gene expression acquired as a part of the biofilm. Therefore, the now planktonic bacteria still possess the same enhanced antibiotic resistance as the parent biofilm and are not susceptible to conventional antibiotics.

An example of a biofilm in the oral cavity is dental plaque. More than 700 bacterial species comprise what we know as "normal oral flora." As most of these bacteria exist as biofilms, they are resistant to antibiotics, as described previously.

In early odontogenic infections, facultative streptococci and anaerobes are most frequently involved, and the specific species have been well-documented.[10] Penicillins are used most often in these infections, as they offer excellent coverage over the susceptible streptococci and other aerobic species involved. As the infection progresses, anaerobes predominate and the effectiveness of penicillin alone is reduced. Adding metronidazole or changing to clindamycin is recommended for better anaerobic coverage. Clindamycin is especially useful for treating odontogenic infections for its excellent bone and abscess penetration and is the preferred antibiotic if the patient is penicillin allergic. If the patient is not responding to complete removal of the infective source, appropriate incision and drainage and empiric antibiotic therapy, then culture and sensitivity testing may provide additional insight into the infective organisms and necessitate an alteration in antibiotic therapy.

Recent international studies have shown that, on average, dentists write at least 2 to 3 prescriptions for antibiotics per week.[11–14] These studies have examined multiple aspects of antibiotic use, including specific drug prescribed, reason for prescribing, and duration of antibiotic therapy. In each of these studies, reasons such as patient demands and lack of updated knowledge of the prescriber have influenced the practitioners' decisions to prescribe antibiotics at least as much as the patients' clinical diagnosis.[15] The results also demonstrated a wide array of prescribing practices with regard to clinical indications, choice of antibiotic, and length of therapy. With regard to duration of therapy, one survey found that the average prescribed course of antibiotics is just fewer than 7 days.[16] An American study showed that endodontists average 8 days for an antibiotic regimen.[17]

Prophylactic administration of oral antibiotics may be indicated in some cases, but the data and literature to support their use are inconsistent. Many recent studies have demonstrated that neither preoperative nor postoperative prophylactic administration of antibiotics have shown any statistically significant benefit with regard to surgical site infection or alveolar osteitis over patients who did not receive antibiotic prophylaxis.[18–21] However, some recent studies have demonstrated a decrease in surgical site infections and pain with prophylactic preoperative administration of antibiotics.[22,23] This argument has continued for decades and likely will persist, given the numerous conflicting reports available. Prophylaxis for patients with certain cardiac conditions and with total-joint prostheses may require antibiotic prophylaxis before some dental procedures. The American Dental Association, American Heart Association, and American Academy of Orthopedic Surgeons have updated their recommendations on the need for prophylaxis based on recent research. Even still, the data that support these practices are also controversial, and clinicians are advised to use their best judgment in the given clinical situation.

Prophylactic antibiotics may be indicated in treatment of the immunocompromised patient as well. Patients with poorly controlled diabetes, chronic steroid users, and patients with immunedeficiency diseases (eg, HIV+) may benefit from preoperative antibiotic prophylaxis before surgical procedures.[24,25] But as mentioned before, preoperative antibiotic prophylaxis in other patients is not supported by current literature.

Pain experienced from pulpitis, periodontitis, alveolar osteitis, or peri-implantitis is not an indication for antibiotics. The antibiotics may serve to decrease local inflammation caused by surface biofilm bacteria and, therefore, reduce the patient's symptoms. These patients require mechanical or surgical intervention in the form of caries control, extractions, root canal therapy, scaling, and root planing, for example, and not systemic antibiotics. Patients presenting with cellulitis or abscess involving fascial planes may benefit from systemic antibiotics, however. In these circumstances, antibiotics serve as an adjunctive measure to surgical or mechanical removal of the infective source that may prevent the hematogenous or local spread of the infective bacteria. These recommendations are summarized in **Table 2**.

Although circumstances exist when systemic antibiotics are indicated, proactive local measures are usually sufficient in treating bacterial infections

Table 2
Recommended treatment of common oral conditions

Operative Intervention	Antibiotics with Operative Intervention
Reversible pulpitis	Lateral periodontal abscess
Irreversible pulpitis	Pericoronitis
Periapical periodontitis	Fascial space infection (cellulitis/abscess)
Alveolar osteitis	Osteomyelitis
Gingivitis	Bisphosphonate-related osteonecrosis of the jaws
Chronic periodontitis	Peri-implantitis

of the oral cavity before antibiotics are truly indicated. Strict adherence to universal precautions and sterile technique when applicable may help prevent disease transmission as well. As dentists, we can do little to limit the use of antibiotics in agriculture or regulate dumping of antibiotic manufacturing by-products into the environment. But we can strive to practice responsible, evidence-based medicine and dentistry.

REFERENCES

1. Wise R, Hart T, Carrs O, et al. Antimicrobial resistance is a major threat to public health. Br Med J 1998;317:609–10.
2. Davies J, Davies D. Origins and evolution of antibiotic resistance. Microbiol Mol Biol Rev 2010;74(3): 417–33.
3. Summary report on antimicrobials sold or distributed for use in food producing animals. Silver Spring (MD): Food and Drug Administration, Department of Health and Human Services; 2009.
4. Mellon M, Benbrook C, Benbrook KL. Hogging it: estimates of antimicrobial abuse in livestock. Washington, DC: Union of Concerned Scientists; 2001.
5. Lipsitch M, Singer R, Levin B. Antibiotics in agriculture: When is it time to close the barn door? Proc Natl Acad Sci U S A 2002;99(9):5752–4.
6. Food and Drug Administration, Center for Veterinary Medicine. The human health impact of fluoroquinolone-resistant campylobacter attributed to the consumption of chicken. Washington, DC: Food Drug Admin; 2001.
7. Smith KE, Besser JM, Hedberg CW, et al. Quinolone-resistant *Campylobacter jejuni* infections in Minnesota, 1992–1998. Investigation team. N Engl J Med 1999;340(20):1525–32.
8. Kinde H, Read DH, Ardans A, et al. Sewage effluent: likely source of *Salmonella enteritidis*, phage type 4 infection in a commercial chicken layer flock in southern California. Avian Dis 1996;40(3):672–6.
9. Fick J, Söderström H, Lindberg RH, et al. Contamination of surface, ground, and drinking water from pharmaceutical production. Environ Toxicol Chem 2009;28(12):2522–7.
10. Flynn T, Halpern L. Antibiotic selection in head and neck infections. Oral Maxillofac Surg Clin North Am 2003;15:17–38.
11. Chate RA, White S, Hale LR, et al. The impact of clinical audit on antibiotic prescribing in general dental practice. Br Dent J 2006;201:635–41.
12. Mainjot A, D'Hoore W, Vanheusden A, et al. Antibiotic prescribing in dental practice in Belgium. Int Endod J 2009;42:1112–7.
13. Dar Odeh NS, Abu-Hammad OA, Al-Omiri MK, et al. Antibiotic prescribing practices by dentists: a review. Ther Clin Risk Manag 2010;6:301–6.
14. Salako N, Rotimi VO, Adib SM, et al. Pattern of antibiotic prescription in the management of oral diseases among dentists in Kuwait. J Dent 2004; 32:503–9.
15. Longman LP, Preston AJ, Martin MV, et al. Endodontics in the adult patient: the role of antibiotics. J Dent 2000;28:539–48.
16. Epstein JB, Chong S, Le ND. A survey of antibiotic use in dentistry. J Am Dent Assoc 2000;131(11): 1600–9.
17. Yingling NM, Byrne BE, Hartwell GR. Antibiotic use by members of the American Association of Endodontists in the year 2000: report of a national survey. J Endod 2002;28(5):396–404.
18. Siddiqi A, Morkel JA, Zafar S. Antibiotic prophylaxis in third molar surgery: a randomized double-blind placebo-controlled clinical trial using split-mouth technique. Int J Oral Maxillofac Surg 2010;39(2): 107–14.
19. Kaczmarzyk T, Wichlinski J, Stypulkowska J, et al. Single-dose and multi-dose clindamycin therapy fails to demonstrate efficacy in preventing infectious and inflammatory complications in third molar surgery. Int J Oral Maxillofac Surg 2007;36(5):417–22.
20. Poeschl PW, Eckel D, Poeschl E. Postoperative prophylactic antibiotic treatment in third molar surgery—a necessity? J Oral Maxillofac Surg 2004; 62(1):3–8.
21. Hill M. No benefit from prophylactic antibiotics in third molar surgery. Evid Based Dent 2005;6(1):10.
22. Halpern LR, Dodson TB. Does prophylactic administration of systemic antibiotics prevent postoperative inflammatory complications after third molar surgery? J Oral Maxillofac Surg 2007;65(2):177–85.
23. Monaco G, Tavernese L, Agostini R, et al. Evaluation of antibiotic prophylaxis in reducing postoperative infection after mandibular third molar extraction in young patients. J Oral Maxillofac Surg 2009;67(7): 1467–72.
24. Termine N, Panzarella V, Ciavarella D, et al. Antibiotic prophylaxis in dentistry and oral surgery: use and misuse. Int Dent J 2009;59(5):263–70.
25. Tong DC, Rothwell BR. Antibiotic prophylaxis in dentistry: a review and practice recommendations. J Am Dent Assoc 2000;131(3):366–74.

How Can We Diagnose and Treat Osteomyelitis of the Jaws as Early as Possible?

Gerard F. Koorbusch, DDS, MBA, FICD[a],*,
Joseph R. Deatherage, DMD, MD[a], Joel K. Curé, MD[b]

KEYWORDS

• Osteomyelitis • Maxilla • Mandible • Jaws

Maxillofacial osteomyelitis is an uncommon condition encountered in the clinical practice of oral and maxillofacial surgery, which presents an enigma for the clinician in terms of diagnosis and treatment. Delayed recognition of the infection may result in a protracted course of treatment and increased surgical morbidity.

The scientific literature is replete with case reports and retrospective studies related to osteomyelitis of the jaws, which do not always give a structured protocol for the early diagnosis and treatment of the disease. The function of this article is to elucidate that structured protocol to enable the timely management of the condition.

Osteomyelitis of the jaws is defined as an inflammatory process of the medullary portion of the affected bone. Osteomyelitis of the jaws is predominantly a disease of the mandible, whereas the maxilla by virtue of its vascularity and thin cortical plates is less frequently involved. In the mandible, the inflammatory process begins with an infection of the medullary portion of the bone and eventually extends to include the haversian systems and the periosteum. Osteomyelitis is truly an infection of bone.[1–4]

Demographically, the infection is more frequently found in the mandible, predominantly in men, with a wide reported age range.[5]

CLASSIFICATION

The focus of this article is the discussion of acute and chronic suppurative osteomyelitis. Acute osteomyelitis is the early phase of the disease, which is usually a suppurative (pus forming) condition.[3] The acute phase may lead to the chronic phase of the disease, which has been arbitrarily defined as osseous infection lasting at least 1 month.[4] Chronic forms of osteomyelitis may be suppurative or nonsuppurative.

Other forms of osteomyelitis of the jawbones include osteoradionecrosis (ORN), bisphosphonate-related osteonecrosis of the jaws (BRONJ), Garrè osteomyelitis, chronic recurrent multifocal osteomyelitis of children, and chronic sclerosing osteomyelitis.

ORN is the death of osseous tissue associated with a radiation injury to the mandible in most cases. This condition is the result of radiation therapy to the maxillofacial region for the treatment of malignant tumors. The tissue injury is represented by a chronic nonhealing wound of the affected jaw, typically with exposure of bone. The progressive radiation injury evolves in chronic hypovascularity, hypocellularity, and ultimately hypoxemia. Cell death and nonhealing osseous lesions ensue. ORN represents avascular necrosis of bone rather than a primary infection of bone.[6]

The authors have nothing to disclose.
[a] Private Practice, Face and Jaw Surgery Center, 1140 West Capitol Avenue, Bismarck, ND 58501, USA
[b] Department of Radiology, University of Alabama at Birmingham, West Pavilion, Room P150, 619 18th Street South, Birmingham, AL 32533, USA
* Corresponding author.
E-mail address: gfkoms@gmail.com

Oral Maxillofacial Surg Clin N Am 23 (2011) 557–567
doi:10.1016/j.coms.2011.07.011
1042-3699/11/$ – see front matter © 2011 Elsevier Inc. All rights reserved.

oralmaxsurgery.theclinics.com

BRONJ is a necrosis of bone related to the long-term use of bisphosphonate drugs. In this condition, the osteoclasts are poisoned by ingestion of the bisphosphonate during normal bone remodeling, resulting in diminished bone loss, which is beneficial in conditions such as osteoporosis. The drugs are also beneficial in the treatment of certain malignancies because they help reduce the spread of the malignancy to bone. Alveolar bone undergoes more rapid bone turnover than skeletal bone; however, in the aftermath of bisphosphonate administration, senescence and death of osteocytes, which cannot be resorbed by osteoclasts, results in necrosis.[7]

Garrè sclerosing osteomyelitis was first described in 1893 and describes an osteomyelitic condition secondary to a proliferative periostitis. The result is a hard swelling of bone often noted in the mandibular first molar region in response to a carious first molar. Radiographs reveal a focal area of cortical-layered thickening, which has been termed onionskin appearance. The disease is usually seen in patients younger than 25 years, and the treatment consists of removal of the offending tooth.[1,2]

Chronic recurrent multifocal osteomyelitis of children refers to a condition characterized by an inflammatory process, which presents with findings similar to infectious osteomyelitis; however, no infectious source is identifiable. The condition affects individuals in their preteenage and teenage years. The disease is polyostotic and may affect the mandible. The treatment is controversial, and the disease may resolve spontaneously.[2]

Chronic diffuse sclerosing osteomyelitis is a condition characterized by an intermedullary osseous infection, which induces the sclerosis. Marx and colleagues[8] demonstrated a bacterial cause for the disease, especially *Actinomyces* species and *Eikenella corrodens.* The disease is predominantly found in women and appears radiographically as medullary sclerosis with little cortical expansion. Inferior alveolar canal widening may occur over time. The disease is often painful in affected patients. The therapy includes antibiotic therapy and surgical debridement. In some refractory cases, hyperbaric oxygen therapy may be indicated.[2,4]

The remainder of this article is devoted to the discussion of acute and chronic suppurative osteomyelitis of the jaws.

ETIOLOGY

Osteomyelitis of the jaws is caused by some inciting focus that enables the infection to propagate. Specific causative factors include odontogenic infection, whether from periodontal disease, periapical abscess, or adjacent soft issue infection; contaminated facial fractures; or foreign bodies such as implants, wires, or bone plates and screws.[2,4,5]

Comorbidities are varied and include malnutrition, alcoholism, substance abuse, smoking, human immunodeficiency virus infection, sickle cell anemia, malignancy, myeloid disorders, hypertension, pulmonary disease, immunosuppression, diabetes mellitus, steroid use, heavy metal toxicity, fibrous dysplasia, Paget disease, and osteopetrosis.[1,2,5,9,10]

CLINICAL FINDINGS

Acute osteomyelitis is characterized by intense pain, swelling that is frequently firm and indurated, fever, paresthesia or anesthesia of the inferior alveolar nerve, and a clearly identifiable cause. Over time, loosening of the teeth, fistula formation transorally or facially, lymphadenopathy, and pathologic fracture may be consequences of the infection.[1-3]

Chronic osteomyelitis has as its primary clinical expression deep pain, fever, malaise, and anorexia. The infection is usually attributable to long-standing odontogenic infection or inadequately treated facial fractures. Once again, loose teeth, intraoral or facial fistula formation, trismus, malocclusion, sequestra, and potentially pathologic fracture may be anticipated. Indurated swelling and lymphadenopathy is often associated with chronic osteomyelitis. Exposure or exfoliation of infected bone fragments may be seen in the course of the disease.[1,2,4]

RADIOLOGIC CONSIDERATIONS

Roles for imaging in maxillofacial osteomyelitis include disease detection and staging, differential diagnosis, and monitoring of treatment response. Because pretherapeutic symptom duration is one of the most significant factors influencing the curability of mandibular osteomyelitis,[11] accurate early diagnosis is critical in the management of maxillofacial osteomyelitis.

Available modalities for imaging evaluation of patients with maxillofacial osteomyelitis include plain and orthopantomographic radiographs, computed tomography (CT), magnetic resonance imaging (MRI), and radionuclide imaging (scintigraphy). Given its frequent odontogenic origin, the initial imaging manifestations of acute osteomyelitis are often observed on plain dental or panorex radiographs. Because they require a loss of up to 50% of bone mineral density to reveal disease, these studies may be normal for up to 8 days or even as long as 3 weeks from symptom onset.[12,13] Radiographic findings in acute osteomyelitis reflect demineralization and destruction of trabeculae within cancellous bone and include ill-defined lucency adjacent to either an extracted tooth socket (**Fig. 1**) or a carious or restored tooth with a lucent periapical inflammatory lesion.[14] Additional findings may include widening of the periodontal ligament space, loss of the lamina dura, and loss of sharp margination (with apparent widening) of the mandibular nerve canal and mental foramen. Subacute findings may include sequestra (radiodense intraosseous necrotic bone fragments) and periosteal new bone formation, but these are often difficult to appreciate on plain radiographs. In chronic suppurative osteomyelitis, plain radiographs demonstrate variably mixed mandibular lucency and sclerosis and bone enlargement related to cortical thickening by appositional periosteal new bone formation.[14]

Radionuclide scintigraphy using 3-phase imaging and technetium Tc 99m (^{99m}Tc)-labeled bisphosphonates demonstrates abnormal radionuclide accumulation in mandibular osteomyelitis because of inflammation and pathologic bone turnover. Findings may be abnormal as early as 2 to 3 days after symptom onset.[15] Early blood flow phase images obtained during the intravenous infusion of radionuclide demonstrate increased uptake as a result of hyperemia in the affected area.[16] Uptake during this blood flow phase is not usually observed in chronic mandibular osteomyelitis.[17] Blood pool phase images (obtained within 5 minutes of the injection) and bone phase images (obtained approximately 3 hours after the blood pool images) demonstrate increased uptake in both acute and chronic osteomyelitis. Uptake on blood pool images reflects altered vascular permeability, whereas persistent uptake on delayed images reflects increased osteoblastic activity at sites of inflammation (**Fig. 2**).

In addition to poor spatial resolution, routine radionuclide bone scans have low specificity,[16] problems that may be mitigated with the addition of single photon emission CT methodology and use of alternative radionuclide agents. Increased uptake on blood flow phase images may be seen with soft tissue infection, and increased uptake on bone phase images occurs in healing fractures, dental extraction, or surgical sites and within osseous neoplasms and other osseous diseases (eg, Paget disease, fibrous dysplasia). Prolonged uptake of radionuclide during bone healing may confound interpretation of radionuclide studies used to monitor treatment. However, decreasing uptake on serial scans correlates with treatment response, whereas renewed uptake signals disease recurrence. Specificity of radionuclide examinations is better (especially in patients with indwelling surgical hardware) when using white blood cells (WBCs) tagged with indium In 111 or ^{99m}Tc hexamethylpropyleneamine oxime (HMPAO).[18] Because WBCs accumulate in normal marrow, the specificity of ^{99m}Tc HMPAO–tagged WBC studies can be improved still further by

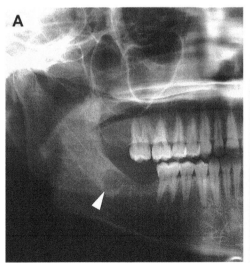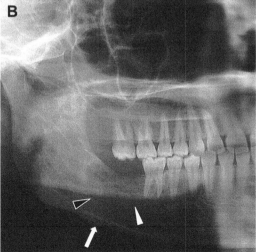

Fig. 1. Subacute suppurative mandibular osteomyelitis after dental extraction. (*A*) Right hemimandible, panorex radiograph. Arrowhead indicates site of persistent pain at tooth number 32 extraction site. Extraction socket and mandibular nerve canal margins are well defined. (*B*) Follow-up panorex image demonstrates diffuse lucency in bone mesial to the extraction site (*white arrowhead*). Margins of the mandibular nerve canal and mesial wall of the extraction socket are now obscure (*outlined arrowhead*). Early periosteal new bone formation is indicated by the white arrow.

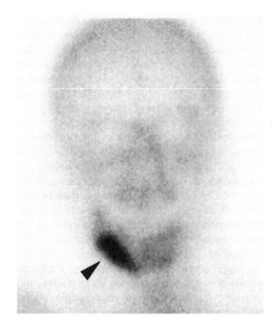

Fig. 2. Right mandibular osteomyelitis on ^{99m}Tc radio-nuclide bone scan (bone phase image, anteroposterior projection). Arrowhead indicates intense uptake in the right mandibular body.

artifacts that adversely affect MRI quality), scintigraphy is an excellent alternative for treatment surveillance. Whole-body radionuclide bone scans are also useful for detection of multifocal involvement in cases of nonsuppurative primary chronic mandibular osteomyelitis associated with systemic diseases known as synovitis, acne, pustulosis, hyperostosis, and osteitis or chronic recurrent multifocal osteomyelitis.

MRI is sensitive for soft tissuepathology but is relatively insensitive for bone and dental pathology. Because of their low mobile proton density, healthy cortical bone, teeth, and sequestra yield weak signal and therefore appear as dark signal voids. Alteration of the normal signal generated by fatty marrow elements in the medullary compartment of the bone is a useful marker for the pathologic condition. Normal fat appears "bright" on T1-weighted (short pulse repetition time, short echo time) MRI. Inflammatory exudate, marrow fibrosis, trabecular thickening, or tumors decrease this marrow signal by altering or replacing normal fat. Short tau inversion recovery MRI depicts tissues with increased water content as bright and nulls signal from fat. This sequence is valuable for demonstrating exudate and edema within bone or in the perimandibular soft tissues, including the subperiosteal and masticator spaces. Contrast-enhanced T1-weighted imaging in conjunction with fat suppression techniques helps define hypervascular tissue in both inflammatory and neoplastic disease. Both abnormal signal and contrast enhancement within the bone and adjacent soft tissues is maximal in acute osteomyelitis and decreases with chronic disease (**Fig. 3**). Contrast

correlation with scans using ^{99m}Tc-labeled nanocolloids that accumulate in normal marrow.[16] In treatment-responsive disease, abnormal uptake on these studies resolves earlier than CT abnormalities. In patients who have contraindications for MRI (eg, cardiac pacemakers or other implanted ferromagnetic materials) or those with surgical hardware in the maxillofacial region (which creates

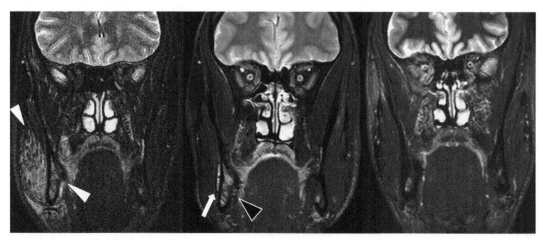

Fig. 3. Right mandibular osteomyelitis on coronal short tau inversion recovery MRI. Images were acquired (from left to right) at presentation, 2 months, and 1-year follow-up. Initial image demonstrates edema in masseter muscle and mandibular medullary compartment (*arrowheads*). On follow-up, soft tissue changes have decreased markedly. There is a persistent high signal in the buccal subperiosteal region (*arrow*) and within the mandible (*outlined arrowhead*). At 1-year follow-up, the findings are essentially normal.

enhancement highlights periosteal/subperiosteal inflammation (**Fig. 4**), which may require surgical resection. MRI demonstrates disease when CT results are negative, demonstrates more extensive disease (including subperiosteal disease) than is depicted by CT, and may more accurately guide debridement.[14] Absence of enhancement helps distinguish osseous sequestra from normal bone. Decreasing enhancement in chronic osteomyelitis probably reflects obliteration of marrow spaces and reduced vascularity of the fibrotic/sclerotic cancellous bone.

Marrow signal changes may take up to 6 months to return to normal after successful therapy. This prolongation limits the usefulness of MRI for treatment monitoring during the first 6 months. However, as with radionuclide examinations, normalization of imaging abnormalities suggests treatment success. After 6 months, MRI is more specific than CT for detecting ongoing infection or recurrence. Interpretation of MRI in patients with osteomyelitis and underlying bone diseases (eg, sickle cell disease) and maxillofacial surgical hardware may be difficult because of abnormal baseline bone appearance and artifacts (**Fig. 5**), respectively.

CT is more sensitive than plain radiographs for subtle early trabecular demineralization in acute osteomyelitis. Maxillofacial CT examinations can be performed with a helical high-resolution CT (HRCT) technique using submillimeter (0.67 mm) slice thickness. Precontrast images are reconstructed in a bone algorithm and viewed in a bone window to optimally depict fine trabecular detail and periosteal new bone formation. Postcontrast images are reconstructed in a soft tissue algorithm and viewed in soft tissue windows that optimize visualization of paramandibular soft tissue swelling and pathologic contrast enhancement (**Fig. 6**). Coronal images are automatically reformatted from the axial data. Additional oblique planes and volume-rendered 3-dimensional images are routinely generated on 3-dimensional workstations. Oblique sagittal and axial images parallel to the mandibular body are very useful for evaluating extension of disease along the mandibular body and evaluating tooth displacement and apical erosion. True coronal imaging oriented perpendicular to the long axis of the mandibular body is useful for evaluating periapical disease, buccolingual extent of disease, sinus tracts, and periosteal new bone formation. These conditions are typically more pronounced along the buccal and lingual surfaces of the mandibular body and angle in which it is difficult to visualize on plain radiographs.

Given its cross-sectional methodology, CT can demonstrate early features of impending cortical perforation (cortical bone thinning) and the full extent of intramedullary disease to better advantage than plain radiographs. Although osseous sequestra and periosteal new bone formation may be detected as early as the third or fourth symptomatic week, these findings are more typically encountered in the chronic phase (>4 weeks) of mandibular osteomyelitis. Cortical interruption is said to be unusual in acute osteomyelitis. However, in the authors' population, cortical interruption is often encountered in patients presenting with acute periapical dental abscesses that have extended into the paramandibular soft tissues. Associated soft tissue abnormalities (masticator space edema, regional adenopathy, abscesses, sinuses, and fistulae) are much better depicted with CT than radiography. Foreign bodies or retained tooth fragments are usually obvious on CT. The severity of swelling and contrast uptake on CT decreases in the chronic phase. Late-developing swelling or increased enhancement of muscles suggests disease recurrence or exacerbation.

On CT, chronic suppurative osteomyelitis is characterized by a mixture of lucency and sclerosis (**Fig. 7**A). Medullary bone sclerosis is characteristic, and its extent correlates with disease duration.[14] Expansion of cortical bone due to periosteal new bone formation may increase the buccolingual width of the bone as well as narrowing of the medullary cavity. Periosteal new bone formation tends to be more prominent in children and adolescents than in adults. Periostitis ossificans is a multilaminated pattern of periosteal

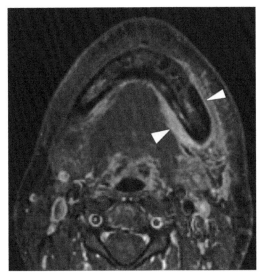

Fig. 4. Left mandibular chronic osteomyelitis. Marked periosteal thickening is well demonstrated on this axial fat-suppressed contrast-enhanced T1-weighted magnetic resonance image (*arrowheads*).

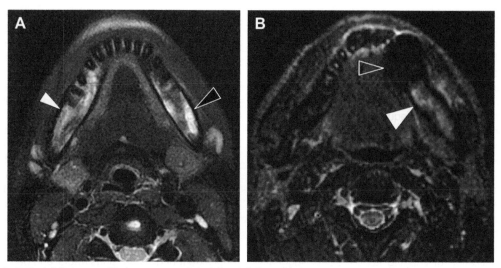

Fig. 5. MRI pitfalls in mandibular osteomyelitis. (*A*) Axial short tau inversion recovery (STIR) image from a patient with sickle cell anemia and recent sickle cell crisis, with right mandibular osteomyelitis. The left hemimandible was clinically normal. The area of infected bone on the right (*solid white arrowhead*) is difficult to distinguish from the baseline abnormal bone on the left (*outlined arrowhead*). (*B*) Axial STIR image shows left mandibular osteomyelitis with metallic hardware in place. Note that the artifacts generated by the hardware obscure the mesial left mandibular body (*outlined arrowhead*). Marrow edema (*solid arrowhead*) is evident distally. The extent of the disease mesially is difficult to evaluate.

new bone formation that is inappropriately connected with Garrè, who never described this process (see **Fig. 7**B). Cortical erosion, sequestrum, and involucrum (periosteal new bone enveloping a sequestrum) formation are commonly encountered on CT in chronic suppurative mandibular osteomyelitis but not with primary nonsuppurative chronic mandibular osteomyelitis. Three CT patterns may be observed in patients with chronic osteomyelitis.[19] These patterns include a bone defect pattern that histologically correlates with fiber-rich granulation tissue, a frosted glass pattern corresponding to formation of tiny osseous trabeculae, and a compact bone pattern that correlates with thickening of osseous trabeculae. CT findings in successfully treated chronic mandibular osteomyelitis may progress from the bone defect pattern to the frosted glass and ultimately compact bone patterns before returning to normal. Conversion of the frosted glass or compact bone pattern to the bone defect pattern in a given area of bone suggests disease recrudescence. These features may be helpful when using CT to monitor treatment of mandibular osteomyelitis, although normalization of CT abnormalities lags behind clinical response. The CT appearance of the mandible in chronic suppurative osteomyelitis eventually returns to normal or near normal. This appearance does not occur in nonsuppurative chronic osteomyelitis (**Fig. 8**). Nonsuppurative

chronic osteomyelitis also lacks CT features of cortical breakthrough and sequestrum formation.

LABORATORY FINDINGS

Patients with acute osteomyelitis may present with leukocytosis or even a normal white cell count, whereas those with chronic osteomyelitis may have a completely normal laboratory profile throughout the course of the disease. Laboratory testing of serum parameters does not frequently aid in the diagnosis and treatment of either form of osteomyelitis.

The microbiology of the facial bone osteomyelitis is consistent with the spectrum of odontogenic infection: polymicrobial.[3,5] Culture and sensitivity testing of specimens from the affected osseous sites may be diagnosed as normal oral flora if the laboratory is not specifically warned of the need for more extensive evaluation of the specimen to determine the spectrum of organisms in the specimen and in directing the administration of appropriate antibiotic therapy.[5] Contemporary laboratory techniques using DNA and RNA identification of microorganisms establish the causative agents of infection more accurately and definitively. Well-analyzed specimens may show predominant organisms and, with antibiotic sensitivity testing, may substantially focus antibiotic therapy to shorten the overall course of the disease.[20]

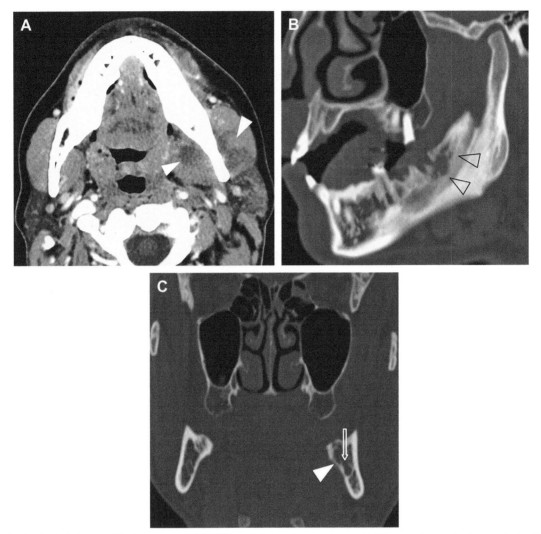

Fig. 6. Acute left mandibular osteomyelitis CT. (*A*) Axial contrast-enhanced CT image demonstrates marked left masticator muscle swelling with masticator space abscesses (*arrowheads*). (*B*) Sagittal oblique image demonstrates mottle lucency distal to the left third molar extraction socket (*arrowheads*). (*C*) True coronal CT image (perpendicular to long axis of mandibular body) demonstrates thinning of the lingual bone (*arrowhead*, compare with the right side) and demineralization of the upper aspect of the mandibular nerve canal (*arrow*).

The histologic findings of acute osteomyelitis show an inflammatory exudate, decreased osteoblasts, and increased osteoclasts. Necrotic bone may present with an acellular histologic picture.[6]

In chronic forms of the disease, chronic inflammatory cells (lymphocytes and plasma cells) may be limited in number and venous thrombosis may be noted. The development of septic thrombi in the mandible may explain the development of paresthesia in some cases. Organisms in the specimen may be difficult to identify, and the histologic findings may be variable.[6]

THE ROLE OF BIOFILMS

Bacteria are found in both planktonic and biofilm varieties. Costerton[20] has defined a biofilm as a "multicellular community composed of prokaryotic and/or eukaryotic cells embedded in a matrix composed, at least partially of material synthesized by sessile cells in the community." The investigator has characterized the biofilm as a combination of bacteria and slime. Bacteria prefer the multicellular lifestyle of the biofilm both in nature and in chronic infections versus the planktonic form, in which the cells have rapid growth and mobility. Planktonic bacteria are more

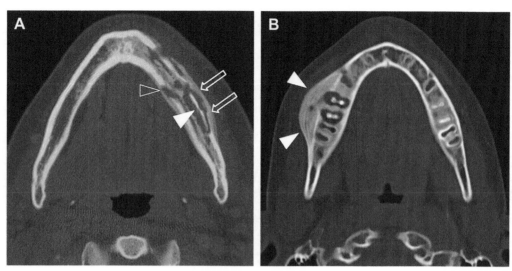

Fig. 7. Chronic suppurative mandibular osteomyelitis CT. (*A*) Axial image demonstrates osseous sequestrum (*solid white arrowhead*), lingual cortical erosion (*outlined arrowhead*), and periosteal new bone/involucrum (*arrows*). (*B*) Right-sided proliferative periostitis. Axial CT image demonstrates lamellated buccal cortical periosteal new bone formation (*arrowheads*) in a child with osteomyelitis caused by actinomycosis.

likely to be expressed in disease states in the form of acute infection and are more susceptible to antibiotic therapy.[20]

Biofilms are not necessarily the cause of infection in all cases and often are not pathogenic.

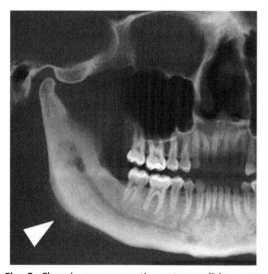

Fig. 8. Chronic nonsuppurative osteomyelitis, panoramic image from cone beam CT examination. Arrowhead indicates thick periosteal new bone formation at the mandibular angle and diffuse osseous sclerosis. Note absence of sequestra. There is a narrowing of the medullary cavity because of marked cortical thickening that extends to involved non–tooth-bearing portions of the mandible, all characteristic of this disease.

However, they have been associated with infections of implantable devices such as artificial joints and mechanical heart valves, indwelling catheters, periodontal disease, root canals, osteomyelitis, prostatitis, endocarditis, and otitis media. When biofilms are the source of infective bacteria, the disease process is disseminated through the release of planktonic bacteria causing the symptoms of acute infection and by inflammation secondary to the biofilm itself involving large areas of the affected tissue.[20] High concentrations of antibiotic agents potentially eradicate the planktonic forms of bacteria but have little effect on the long-term viability of the biofilm, which is highly resistant to antibiotics.[20] To effectively treat an infection in bone caused by a biofilm, surgical removal of all affected bone has been demonstrated as the method of choice.[20] Treatment with antibiotic therapy alone may lead to continuing osseous destruction during repeated therapeutic cycles, which may reduce the patient's symptoms but result in overall treatment failure.[20]

TREATMENT

The standard surgical treatment regimen for osteomyelitis has been well established in the scientific literature. These principles remain as applicable today as they did when initially presented, and they may be summarized as follows:

1. Early diagnosis
2. Elimination of the source of the infection
3. Establishment of surgical drainage

4. Bacteriologic identification and antibiotic sensitivity testing
5. Appropriate antibiotic coverage
6. Surgical debridement
7. Supportive care
8. Reconstruction.

The early diagnosis of osteomyelitis of the jaws is often predicated on the clinical suspicion of the treating surgeon. A high index of suspicion coupled with a thorough clinical examination and appropriate imaging leads the clinician to the presumptive diagnosis. The establishment of surgical drainage by transoral or extraoral exploration enables the surgeon to obtain material for bacterial identification and antibiotic sensitivity testing, as well as removal of any pockets of purulence and visual inspection of the extent of the disease.

Antibiotic administration should always be instituted after bacterial identification and sensitivity testing; however, delays in treatment should be avoided. This dilemma may be circumvented by the administration of penicillin with metronidazole or clindamycin initially until bacterial identification is available. Previous studies have shown that the polymicrobial nature of osteomyelitis presents with a microflora spectrum that is very responsive to the therapeutic regimens normally used to treat odontogenic infections.[2,5] It is important for the clinician to request identification of as many organisms as possible on the submitted specimens to determine the microbial mix of the infection and thus select the most appropriate antibiotic regimen for the patient. Consultation with an infectious disease consultant is often helpful in cases of osteomyelitis to aid identification of the causative organisms and selection of an appropriate antibiotic therapeutic regimen.

Surgical debridement of the osteomyelitic jaw may encompass a series of procedures. The removal of infected and devitalized teeth and associated soft tissue is a preliminary treatment of osteomyelitis, as is the stabilization of fractures with intermaxillary or external pin fixation and the removal of any involved implants or hardware.[6] Internal rigid fixation of fractures during the early treatment of osteomyelitis is not recommended.[6] The removal of necrotic and chronically infected bone is essential to the successful management of the infection. Multiple procedures over a period of days or weeks may be required to eradicate the infection from the affected jaw. The procedures include sequestrectomy, saucerization, decortication, resection, and reconstruction.

Sequestrectomy is the removal of infected devitalized bony fragments in the infected area of the jaw. The sequestrum is often surrounded by a sheath or membrane of new bone, termed an involucrum. The removal of sequestra is important because it enables the penetration of high concentrations of antibiotics into an area of previously poor vascularity. Saucerization is frequently performed in conjunction with sequestrectomy. This procedure removes the margins of necrotic bone to expose the medullary spaces for further exploration and removal of necrotic tissue. The procedure is usually performed intraorally, giving direct access to the infected bone. After the procedure the wound may be packed open to allow irrigation and examination during the early healing of the defect. Once a bed of healthy granulation tissue is formed, the packing may be removed.[1,2]

Decortication is the removal of lateral and inferior cortical plates of bone to gain access to the infected medullary cavity. Avascular bone is removed until a 1- to 2-cm margin of vital bone is achieved.[1] Besides removing devitalized bone and soft tissue, decortication also has the theoretical advantage of shortening the time of antibiotic therapy and decreases the risk of further formation of sequestra and abscesses.[2] This procedure is usually reserved for refractory osteomyelitis that is nonresponsive to more surgically conservative procedures.

Persistent chronic osteomyelitis may require resection with bony margins prepared for immediate or delayed reconstruction. Long-term osteomyelitic infections may lead to pathologic fractures, continuing infection after decortication, or persistent nonunion of facial fractures. In such cases, resection and eventual reconstruction may be indicated to eradicate the disease. The resection margins should be in a viable bone 1 to 2 cm from the site of infection. Reconstruction bone plates or external pin fixation may be placed where prolonged infection or lack of a viable tissue bed precludes bone grafting in the short run.

In severe long-standing refractory cases of osteomyelitis, hyperbaric oxygen therapy may be indicated. In such cases, surgical debridement has been achieved, antibiotic therapy has been directed by bacterial identification and antibiotic sensitivity testing, and no further focus of infection has been identified. The protocol is well identified in the literature.[4]

SPECIAL INFECTIONS

Actinomycosis is a rare infection of the oral-cervicofacial region, which routinely involves both the soft tissue of the area and the mandible. The organisms have characteristics of both bacteria and fungi but require treatment with antibiotics and not antifungal agents. *Actinomyces* species are gram-positive, microaerophilic, non–acid-fast, non–spore-forming bacteria that are normal inhabitants of the mouth. The oral-cervicofacial form of the infection presents with a firm brawny swelling or mass usually associated with a dental extraction or fracture. Rarely the disease may present in the maxilla. The infectious lesion may be painful and is often a red to purple color. Facial fistulae are common, and lymphadenopathy is a late finding. Trismus, periosteal involvement, bony destruction, and drainage of sulfur granules from the fistulae are common. These sulfur granules represent clumps of bacterial colonies when viewed microscopically.[1,2]

The treatment of the disease is consistent with that previously presented for osteomyelitis with the following exceptions: identification of the organism may be difficult and the patient will require long-term antibiotic therapy. Antibiotic therapy includes several weeks of intravenous antibiotics followed by months of orally administered drugs to assure control of the infection. Specific antibiotic regimens have included penicillin, doxycycline, or ceftriaxone.

Nocardia species occasionally cause infection in the head and neck. The organism is not normally an inhabitant of the mouth and usually gains access to the body via inhalation. Nocardia is primarily a pulmonary disease but may spread hematogenously to virtually any organ system. The disease may be encountered in immunocompromised patients. Nocardiosis is very similar in its disease picture to actinomycosis. Chronic infections may present with fistulae, brawny swelling, pain, and limited constitutional symptoms. Surgical management is with debridement and drainage of all abscesses. Identification of the organism is significant because antibiotic therapy with sulfonamides for extended periods of time is recommended in contradistinction to the treatment regimen for actinomycosis.[1,2]

A NEW PARADIGM FOR THE MANAGEMENT OF MAXILLOMANDIBULAR OSTEOMYELITIS

The early diagnosis of osteomyelitis, especially in its chronic forms, is key to the establishment of antibiotic therapy and appropriate surgical intervention. Clinical findings suggestive of osteomyelitis along with a high index of diagnostic suspicion on the part of the treating surgeon are the first step in the treatment path of the disease.

Orthopantomographic imaging will undoubtedly offer some information in the diagnostic process. More definitive imaging can be used, such as scintigraphy, MRI, and CT, but which one is the best? Scintigraphy and MRI are both sensitive but nonspecific. The imaging technique with the best combination of sensitivity and specificity seems to be CT (HRCT). Comparative studies of the various modalities are not currently available.

Laboratory identification and antibiotic sensitivity testing help in directed medical care of the infection. Although a histopathologic diagnosis of osteomyelitis may be confirmatory, it is not in itself usually an early aid to the diagnosis of the disease.[5]

Surgical intervention should be early and aggressive. Multiple surgical procedures may be required to remove all devitalized bone and necrotic soft tissue at the affected site. The early removal of foreign bodies (bone plates, screws, implants) is essential in view of the contemporary concepts of the role of biofilms in infection.

Although the knowledge base, technical expertise, and availability of advanced imaging have increased, suppurative osteomyelitis of the jaws remains a surgical disease and surgical treatment modalities are virtually unchanged in recent decades.

It is the clinical expertise of the surgeon using the clinical signs and symptoms presented, aided with appropriate imaging (HRCT), that result in the early diagnosis of osteomyelitis. Surgical intervention will then enable the surgeon to harvest material for histopathologic diagnosis and bacterial identification. Antibiotic sensitivity testing helps in the selection of the appropriate therapeutic agent, whereas serial imaging may be required to monitor the response of the patient to treatment and help determine its end point.

REFERENCES

1. Koorbusch GF. Infections of the orofacial region. In: Zambito RF, Cleri DJ, editors. Immunology and infectious diseases of the mouth, head and neck. St Louis (MO): Mosby Year Book; 1991. p. 334–41.
2. Topazian RG. Osteomyelitis of the jaws. In: Topazian RG, Goldberg MH, Hupp JR, editors. Oral and maxillofacial infections. 4th edition. Philadelphia: W.B. Saunders Company; 2002. p. 214–42.
3. Mercuri LG. Acute osteomyelitis of the jaws. Oral Maxillofac Surg Clin North Am 1991;3(2):355–65.
4. Marx RE. Acute osteomyelitis of the jaws. Oral Maxillofac Surg Clin North Am 1991;3(2):367–81.
5. Koorbusch GF, Fotos P, Terhark-Goll K. Retrospective assessment of osteomyelitis: etiology, demographics, risk factors, and management in 35 cases. Oral Surg Oral Med Oral Pathol 1992;74(2):149–54.
6. Marx RE, Stern D. Oral & maxillofacial pathology: a rationale for diagnosis and treatment. Carol Stream (IL): Quintessence Publishing Company, Inc; 2003. p. 54–7, 388–94.

7. Marx RE. Oral and intravenous bisphosphonate-induced osteonecrosis of the jaws. Hanover Park (IL): Quintessence Publishing Company, Inc; 2007.

8. Marx RE, Carlson ER, Smith BR, et al. Isolation of a Actinomyces species and Eikenella corrodens from patients with chronic diffuse sclerosing osteomyelitis. J Oral Maxillofac Surg 1994;51:26–33.

9. Hudson JW. Osteomyelitis of the jaws: a 50 year perspective. J Oral Maxillofac Surg 1993;51:1294–301.

10. Veaeau PJ, Koorbusch GF, Finkelstein M. Invasive squamous cell carcinoma of the mandible presenting as a chronic osteomyelitis. J Oral Maxillofac Surg 1990;48:1118–22.

11. Ida M, Watanabe H, Tetsumura A, et al. CT findings as a significant predictive factor for the curability of mandibular osteomyelitis: a multivariate analysis. Dentomaxillofac Radiol 2005;34:86–90.

12. Worth HM, Stonemen DW. Osteomyelitis, malignant disease and fibrous dysplasia. Some radiographic similarities and differences. Dent Radiogr Photogr 1977;50:1–9.

13. Davies HT, Carr RJ. Osteomyelitis of the mandible: a complication of routine dental extractions in the alcoholic. Br J Oral Maxillofac Surg 1990;28:185–8.

14. Schuknecht B, Valavanis A. Osteomyelitis of the mandible. Neuroimaging Clin N Am 2003;13:605–18.

15. Reinert S, Widlitzik H, Venderink DJ. The value of magnetic resonance imaging in the diagnosis of mandibular osteomyelitis. Br J Oral Maxillofac Surg 1999;37:459–63.

16. Gotthardt M, Bleeker-Rovers CP, Boerman OC, et al. Imaging of inflammation by PET, conventional scintigraphy and other imaging techniques. J Nucl Med 2010;51(12):1937–49.

17. Fukmitsu N, Utigawa K, Mori Y, et al. What can be identified by three phase bone scintigraphy in patients with chronic osteomyelitis of the mandible? Ann Nucl Med 2010;24:287–93.

18. Weon YC, Yang S, Choi Y, et al. Use of Tc-99m HMPAO leukocyte scans to evaluate bone infection: incremental value of additional SPECT images. Clin Nucl Med 2000;25(7):519–26.

19. Tanaka R, Hagashi T. Computed tomographic findings of chronic osteomyelitis involving the mandible: correlation to histopathologic findings. Dentomaxillofac Radiol 2008;37:94–103.

20. Costerton W. The biofilm primer. Berlin: Springer-Verlag; 2007. p. 129–80.

Do Dental Infections Really Cause Central Nervous System Infections?

Stewart K. Lazow, MD, DDS[a],*, Steven R. Izzo, DDS[b],
David Vazquez, DMD[b]

KEYWORDS

- Cavernous sinus thrombosis • Brain abscess • Dental
- Odontogenic

In the post–World War I antibiotic era, the prevalence of central nervous system (CNS) infection is estimated to be 1 per 100,000 population.[1] The literature is replete with anecdotal case reports of CNS infections of apparent dental etiology. Conversely, it is widely cited that the incidence of CNS infection of dental etiology is only in the range of 1% to 2%.[2]

Before attempting to answer the question if dental infections really cause CNS infections, we define CNS infection as a condition that includes meningitis, subdural empyema, cerebritis, encephalitis, septic thrombophlebitis, and brain abscess.

Acute bacterial meningitis (viral, tuberculous, parasitic; fungal not included in this discussion of dental etiology) is the immediate effect of bacteria in the subarachnoid space causing an inflammatory reaction in the pia mater and arachnoid as well as in the cerebrospinal fluid (CSF). The large-scale inflammation of meningitis is secondary to the bacterial invasion as well as the immune reaction. The immune response is trifold, resulting in vasogenic cerebral edema, interstitial edema, and cytotoxic edema.

Subdural empyema is an intracranial suppurative process between the inner surface of the dura mater and the outer surface of the arachnoid. This condition is more common in men than women, a feature for which there is little explanation.

Subdural empyema usually originates in the frontal and sphenoid sinuses to the frontal lobe or in the mastoid air cells to the temporal lobe. A collection of subdural pus may range up to 200 mL. This collection may be visualized on computed tomography (CT) with increased meningeal enhancement.

Encephalitis is an acute inflammation of the brain. Encephalitis with meningeal involvement is known as meningoencephalitis. Although usually viral, bacterial and parasitic forms are common in immunocompromised patients. Typical neurologic signs and symptoms include fever, headache, nausea, vomiting, delirium, and seizures. CT or magnetic resonance imaging (MRI) may not be diagnostic. On lumbar puncture, the CSF contains elevated protein level, normal glucose level, numerous white blood cells, and antibodies to the offending organism.

Cerebritis is an inflammation of the cerebrum. It is a focal nonencapsulated purulent infection of the brain parenchyma or immature brain abscess. Cerebritis is characterized by vascular congestion, edema, petechial hemorrhages, and cerebral softening. This condition is ill defined on contrast-enhanced CT scan; it presents with an irregular nonhomogeneous central area of low intensity with mass effect and peripheral enhancement in the form of an incompletely formed ring. MRI is

[a] Department of Dental/Oral and Maxillofacial Surgery, Kings County Hospital Center-SUNY Brooklyn, 451 Clarkson Avenue, Brooklyn, NY, USA
[b] Department of Dental/Oral and Maxillofacial Surgery, Kings County Hospital Center, 451 Clarkson Avenue, Brooklyn, NY, USA
* Corresponding author. University Hospital #76, 445 Lenox Road, Brooklyn, NY 11203.
E-mail address: skloms@aol.com

Oral Maxillofacial Surg Clin N Am 23 (2011) 569–578
doi:10.1016/j.coms.2011.08.001

actually more sensitive than CT in the early cerebritis stage. If untreated, cerebritis will proceed to a brain abscess in 1 to 2 weeks.

Haymaker,[3] in his classic 1945 Army Institute of Pathology review of 28 fatal CNS infections after tooth extraction, cited 4 cases of meningitis, 3 cases of subdural empyema, and 1 case of encephalitis of dental etiology. Since 1945 in the postantibiotic era, the literature is largely devoid of these types of CNS infections of dental etiology.

Therefore, this article focuses on brain abscess and septic cavernous sinus thrombophlebitis of dental etiology.

CAVERNOUS SINUS THROMBOSIS

The dural sinuses drain blood from the brain ultimately into the internal jugular veins. The largest ones involved in septic thrombophlebitis are the superior sagittal sinus, lateral (transverse) sinus, straight sinus, and cavernous sinus. The cavernous sinus is the intracranial sinus most often implicated in dental or odontogenic infection.

The cavernous sinus is, in fact, a bilateral sinus cavity bordered by the temporal and sphenoid bones lateral to the sella turcica (**Fig. 1**). It receives blood from the superior and inferior ophthalmic veins, as well as the sphenoparietal sinus, superficial middle cerebral vein, and pterygoid plexus of veins. The cavernous sinus drains predominantly into the superior and inferior petrosal sinuses and ultimately into the internal jugular vein as well as the emissary veins passing through various cranial foramina.

Contents of the cavernous sinus include cranial nerves III, IV, V_1, V_2, and VI and internal carotid artery (**Fig. 2**). In fact, the cavernous sinus is the only place in the body where an artery travels completely through a venous structure. The abducens nerve passes below the sphenopetrous ligament, which forms a narrow fibrous canal, Dorello canal. Cranial nerve VI then runs with the internal carotid artery in the lateral wall of the cavernous sinus. Therefore, abducens nerve palsy is usually the first cranial nerve injury seen in cavernous sinus thrombosis (CST).

CST, or, more to the point, septic thrombophlebitis, implies an infected blood clot in the cavernous sinus. The patient with CST may present with high fever, headache, photophobia, nausea, vomiting, and signs of systemic toxicity. Obstruction of the ophthalmic veins leads to chemosis, proptosis, and edema of the ipsilateral eyelids, forehead, and nose. Engorgement of the retinal veins may be followed by retinal hemorrhages, papilledema, eye pain, and decreased visual acuity. Cranial nerve involvement (III, IV, V_1, VI) leads to ptosis, ophthalmoplegia, and supraorbital paresthesia. Within 24 to 48 hours, spread of the clot through the circular sinus to the contralateral cavernous sinus may result in bilateral signs and symptoms.

The cause of CST is 2-fold: hematogenous spread of septic emboli to the cavernous sinus via the blood supply of the head and neck or by direct extension of contiguous space infections. Most cases of CST are secondary to infections of the paranasal sinuses (ethmoid, sphenoid, frontal), nasal cavity, tonsils, middle ear, orbit, skin of the nose and face, or teeth.

Predisposing conditions to CST are similar to those for all CNS infections. These conditions include previous head trauma, particularly penetrating cranial injuries, even after intracranial neurosurgical procedures. Immunocompromised patients, including transplant recipients on immunosuppressive medications, patients with cancer on chemotherapy, and human immunodeficiency virus (HIV)-positive patients, are all at increased risk for CNS infection. Patients with nonoperated congenital cardiac cyanotic malfunctions are at increased risk for CNS infection due to septic emboli passing through a right-to-left shunt, bypassing the pulmonary filter. The same mechanism is seen in patients with hereditary hemorrhagic telangiectasia and pulmonary arteriovenous fistulas. Septic embolization from bacterial endocarditis or pulmonary embolism from tuberculosis or pneumonia increases the risk of CNS infection.

The 2 predominant pathogens in reported cases of CST are *Staphylococcus aureus* (50%–60%) and β-hemolytic streptococcus (20%), followed

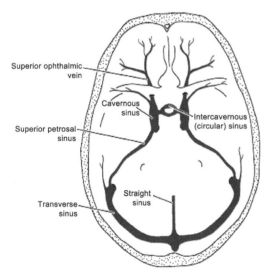

Fig. 1. Axial view of the cavernous sinus.

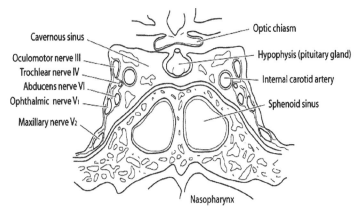

Fig. 2. Coronal view of the contents of the cavernous sinus.

by *Streptococcus pneumoniae*, *Haemophilus influenzae*, and *Bacteroides*. Mucormycosis and *Aspergillus* infections may be seen in those with uncontrolled diabetes. Polymicrobial infections are becoming more frequently diagnosed because of improvement in modern sampling techniques.

It is well known that infection may spread to the cavernous sinus via an anterior or posterior hematogenous pathway. The anterior route involves a retrograde septic thrombophlebitis of the valveless veins coursing through the infraorbital or canine space from the anterior facial vein to the angular vein to the inferior ophthalmic vein through the superior orbital fissure into the cavernous sinus. These valveless veins may drain infections originating from anterior facial structures such as anterior maxillary teeth, skin of the external nose, upper lip, cheek or eyelids, and orbit.

The posterior pathway typically involves infratemporal space infections that may pass via emissary veins from the pterygoid venous plexus through the pterygopalatine fossa to the inferior petrosal sinus into the cavernous sinus or via emissary veins passing through the foramina ovale, lacerum, or Vesalii. Typically these infections arise from maxillary molar teeth, paranasal sinuses, middle ear, or mastoids.

A third pathway of infection to the cavernous sinus is direct extension from an anatomically contiguous focus, such as the paranasal sinuses, middle ear, and mastoids, or orofacial infections spreading along fascial planes to the skull base. Infections of maxillary molars may spread though the maxillary sinus and posterior orbit forming a sphenoid osteomyelitis, which may then extend into the cavernous sinus. Infections of mandibular molars may pass in a submasseteric plane to the infratemporal fossa leading to a temporal bone osteomyelitis or via diploic veins to the cavernous sinus.

After review of the 2 largest early series of CST of apparent dental etiology, namely, those by Haymaker[3] and Childs and Courville,[4] in addition to the more recent anecdotal reports, the following demographics are clear: men outnumber women (2:1), left-sided dental infections outnumber right (3:2), mandibular teeth are more often involved than maxillary teeth (1.5:1), molar teeth from either jaw are involved more than anterior teeth (4:1). The posterior route through the pterygoid plexus is implicated 80% of the time with maxillary or mandibular molars and the anterior retrograde route through the facial vein to the angular vein only 20% of the time, secondary to infection of the maxillary incisors, canines, and first bicuspids.

CT, even with intravenous contrast, shows negative results in up to 25% of patients with diagnosed CST; yet, it remains a useful first-line investigation (**Fig. 3**). Specific changes seen with cerebral venous thrombosis include the empty delta sign, a triangular pattern of enhancement from dilated venous collateral channels surrounding a central relatively hypodense thrombus. Another change is the cord sign seen on a single slice only on non–contrast-enhanced CT scans, in which the fresh thrombus appears as increased density relative to gray matter in structures parallel to the scanning plane.

MRI has greater sensitivity than CT for the changes of central venous thrombosis. In the acute phase at days 3 to 5, the thrombus is isointense on both T1- and T2-weighted sequences. Subsequently, the thrombus becomes hyperintense. After 2 to 3 weeks, bilateral deep hemorrhagic infarcts may be seen.

Cerebral angiography (**Fig. 4**) with late venous views sets the gold standard in the diagnosis of CST. Because of the morbidity and poor patient acceptance, this technique should only be

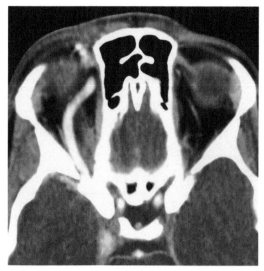

Fig. 3. Contrast-enhanced axial CT shows dilated right superior ophthalmic vein and enlarged ipsilateral cavernous sinus. (*Courtesy of* Amirsys Publishing, Inc, Salt Lake City, UT, USA; with permission.)

performed in those cases in which the diagnosis remains in doubt after MRI. MRI remains the routine standard of diagnostic care.

In the preantibiotic era, septic CST was almost always fatal, with mortality rates approaching 100%. Currently, the mortality rate remains in the range of 20% to 30%.[5] Of those who survive, more than 50% have residual deficits, including blindness, cranial nerve palsy, oculomotor weakness, and pituitary insufficiency.

Treatment of septic CST must be prompt and targeted. The primary infection must be aggressively drained and the cause eradicated. High-dose intravenous antibiotics that cross the blood-brain barrier and are empirically effective against coagulase-positive staphylococcus and streptococcus are indicated. Nafcillin, third-generation cephalosporins such as cefotaxime, and chloramphenicol are appropriate, pending culture and sensitivity results.

The role of anticoagulation in the management of septic CST remains controversial. Advocates of anticoagulant therapy recommend intravenous heparin in line with guidelines for venous thromboembolism. This administration of heparin may prevent extension of the clot into neighboring sinuses and dissemination of septic emboli. Opponents state that anticoagulation aggravates hemorrhagic lesions in the orbit and brain and that the clot itself limits the infection. Thrombolytic infusion has been cited in individual anecdotal cases, but it should be reserved for patients who continue to deteriorate despite antibiotics, anticoagulation, and supportive care.

The role of corticosteroids in CST is less controversial. The use of high-dose steroids to reduce cerebral inflammation and lower intracranial pressure is universally accepted. Steroids may also prevent vascular collapse resulting from pituitary dysfunction.

Adjuvant hyperbaric oxygen (HBO) has not been proven to be effective in the treatment of CST. Neurosurgical drainage or thrombectomy is rarely performed because of technical difficulty and associated grave morbidity.

Before the end of World War II, the literature is replete with cases of CST of dental etiology. In their classic 1942 article, Childs and Courville[4] reported on an astonishing 59 cases of CST secondary to dental infection. In his benchmark 1945 article, Haymaker[3] reported 11 cases of fatal septic cerebral sinus thrombosis after tooth extraction; specifically 9 of these 11 cases were CST.

At the Army Institute of Pathology, Haymaker had the distinct advantage of postmortem examination of the patients to confirm the dental etiology in these 9 cases. Of the 9 cases, 7 were secondary to hematogenous spread of the dental infection. Haymaker was able to identify the most frequent causative pathogen of CST secondary to hematogenous spread as *Streptococcus viridans*. In 2 such cases, the investigator was able to culture

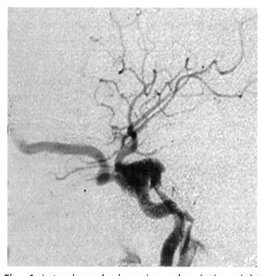

Fig. 4. Lateral cerebral angiography during right internal carotid artery injection shows contrast filling the cavernous sinus and retrograde flow distending the superior ophthalmic vein. (*Courtesy of* Amirsys Publishing, Inc, Salt Lake City, UT, USA; with permission.)

identical streptococci from both the CST and oral cavity, positively confirming the dental etiology. In the cases of direct contiguous spread, *S aureus* was the primary organism cultured from the oral cavity and CST. Osteomyelitis of the greater wing of the sphenoid bone was one of the most striking pathologic features at autopsy.

Since 1945, the number of cases of CST of dental etiology in the scientific literature remains in single digits.[6-9] Careful analysis of 4 of these cases raises several questions regarding the true etiology. Harbour and colleagues[10] reported a fatal case of septic CST associated with gingivitis and parapharyngeal abscess. In this case, a healthy 29-year-old man visited his dentist for pain in the right lower tooth 10 days before admission. The patient's local gingival tenderness responded to a topical anesthetic. On admission, the patient presented with a parapharyngeal abscess and developed CST. Blood cultures were positive for α-hemolytic streptococci, and the parapharyngeal abscess yielded *Bacteroides melaninogenicus* and fusiform bacteria, the most frequent pathogens implicated in neck abscess of odontogenic origin. However at autopsy, the patient's oral cavity showed no sign of dental or gingival infection. The offending bacteria were never cultured from the presumed gingivitis.

Feldman and colleagues[11] reported a case of CST complicating an odontogenic parapharyngeal abscess. A 69-year-old man presented with a bilateral CST and a right parapharyngeal abscess 6 days after receiving a prescription for penicillin from his dentist for a dental abscess. Ultimately, the patient underwent tracheotomy, incision and drainage of the parapharyngeal abscess, and extraction of tooth number 32. The patient responded well to intravenous antibiotics and anticoagulation. Cultures of the parapharyngeal abscess were positive for *Pseudomonas* and diphtheroids, not typical odontogenic bacteria. No culture sample was taken from the extraction site. There was no mention of submandibular, sublingual, pterygomandibular space involvement on CT, which confirmed the parapharyngeal abscess. The parapharyngeal abscess probably spread via the pterygoid plexus of veins to the cavernous sinus. However, it is presumptive to conclude that tooth number 32 caused the parapharyngeal abscess.

Colbert and colleagues[12] reported a case of septic CST and dental infection. A 49-year-old man presented with signs and symptoms consistent with a left CST and poor dentition with apical periodontitis associated with tooth number 16 on panoramic radiograph. No mention was made of purulent drainage or culture report. This condition is at best a presumptive diagnosis of bacteremia secondary to periodontitis that caused hematogenous spread to the cavernous sinus.

Ogundiya and colleagues[13] presented the most convincing case of CST and blindness as complications of an odontogenic infection. A 35-year-old woman presented with signs and symptoms consistent with left CST 11 days after extraction of tooth number 16. She presented with a left temporal space abscess and a left postseptal orbital abscess causing new-onset blindness. Culture results from the posterior maxilla showed rare β-hemolytic streptococci, and culture results from the posterior orbit showed α-hemolytic streptococci and mixed anaerobes. Arteriogram showed a filling defect of the internal carotid artery in the left cavernous sinus, confirming suspicion of the CST. Presumably this case manifests an anterior retrograde pathway to the CST. However, even the investigators admitted the difficulty distinguishing between a postseptal orbital cellulitis, orbital apex syndrome, and CST because these conditions may evolve into one another.

The only way to reliably confirm the dental etiology of CST is via matching culture results of intracranial/extracranial sites of infection. Accurate sensitive culture samples of the oral nidus of infection must be taken and compared with those of the septic CST. An array of molecular fingerprinting techniques based on nucleotide sequencing may now be applied to provide supportive evidence for the identification of isolates from multiple sources. These techniques include biotyping, serotyping, DNA hybridization, and ribosomal RNA sequencing. However, short of postmortem examination, this culturing may be impractical because of the technical difficulty in gaining surgical access to the cavernous sinus. Even fine-needle aspiration or stereotactic biopsy of the cavernous sinus is fraught with complications.

A convincing argument attributing septic CST to odontogenic etiology must satisfy 3 or more of the following conditions:

1. Confirm the diagnosis of CST by clinical presentation and imaging
2. Precisely match the isolated pathogens from intracranial/extracranial sites with identical DNA homology
3. Document a plausible pathway of hematogenous spread of infection
4. Show anatomic evidence of contiguous spread of infection.

Otherwise the diagnosis of CST of dental etiology remains one of exclusion and is not evidence-based.

BRAIN ABSCESS

Brain abscess, which occurs at a rate of 1 per 100,000 population,[14] has often been attributed to dental infection or treatment. A review of the literature reveals numerous cases implicating a dental focus, even though a culture match between the brain and oral focus was not made or the microorganism cultured from the brain was not representative of normal oral flora. There are 3 modes of inoculation: direct contamination through a traumatic or surgical event, hematogenous spread, and spread from a contiguous focus. Extension of orofacial infection can involve the neck, mediastinum, orbit, and cranium. However, because of antibiotics, improved diagnostic imaging techniques, and physicians' diligence in treating maxillofacial infections, these often life-threatening sequelae are not the norm. The diagnosis of brain abscess as a direct result of dental infection has historically been one of exclusion, with some cases being attributed to dental infection simply because there was a dental focus or treatment preceding the development of the abscess. This raises the question if orofacial infections really have the capability of spreading intracranially, ultimately causing brain abscess.

Signs and symptoms of brain abscess are similar to those of any space-occupying lesion. Increased intracranial pressure leads to headache, nausea, and papilledema. The first and most common symptom seen is headache, involving 75% of cases.[15] With progression of the infection, nausea and vomiting are seen and are usually associated with abscesses involving the cerebellum and brainstem. Seizure activity is often the warning sign that leads the patient to seek treatment. However, seizures are only seen about 25% of the time. Fever is seen in only 50% of patients and is usually low grade. Mental status changes and focal neurologic deficits, such as confusion, stupor, ataxia, aphasia, hemiparesis, visual field defects, and sensory disturbances, are seen at about the same frequency (65%), and the type of deficit seen provides a most likely location of the abscess. Aphasia and visual defects indicate a temporal lobe abscess. Frontal lobe abscess manifests drowsiness, motor speech disorder, hemiparesis, and grand mal seizures. Ataxia results from a cerebellar abscess, and dysphagia and facial weakness are seen in brainstem involvement. The classic triad of fever, headache, and focal neurologic deficit is seen in less than half of the cases.

Imaging studies play a vital role in the diagnostic process. Before the introduction of CT scanning, radionuclide brain scans were used, which reveal an area of increased uptake with a cold center (donut sign). Cerebral angiography only suggests a mass lesion if there was displacement of major vessels. The advent of CT scanning has rendered radionuclide brain scans, ventriculography, angiography, and pneumoencephalography nearly obsolete and improved the early diagnosis and localization of brain abscess. Development of brain abscess begins with cerebritis, characterized by cerebral softening, petechial hemorrhages, edema, and vascular congestion. CT performed at this time reveals merely an irregular area of low density with mass effect. With contrast enhancement, an incomplete ring is seen. Once the abscess matures, a postcontrast CT reveals a central area of low density surrounded by a peripherally enhanced ring (**Fig. 5**).[16] Information including the location, size, and number of abscesses as well as progression of treatment can be obtained from CT. The presence of air indicates previous surgical intervention, infection by gas-forming organisms, or the presence of a fistulous tract from extension of an extracranial focus. Some investigators prefer MRI to diagnose brain abscess. MRI findings also depend on the stage of infection at the time of imaging. Cerebritis again is seen as an ill-defined hypointense area on T1-weighted images, whereas T2-weighted images show high signal intensity from the inflammatory infiltrate centrally and peripherally. MRI is actually more sensitive than CT in the early stages because of alterations in tissue water content. As the abscess matures, the proteinaceous necrotic fluid center exhibits higher signal intensity than that of CSF. Once formed, the abscess capsule stands out as a hyperintense ring surrounding the

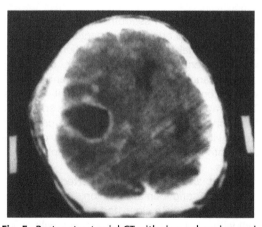

Fig. 5. Postcontrast axial CT with ring-enhancing parietal lobe abscess. (*From* Lazow SK, Kim D. Imaging head and neck infections. Oral and Maxillofac Surg Clin North Am 2001;13:586; with permission.)

hypointense necrotic center on T1-weighted images (**Fig.** 6A). On T2-weighted images, the reverse is seen: a hypointense ring surrounding increased signal density of the necrotic core (see **Fig.** 6B). Gadolinium contrast enhancement produces T1-weighted ring enhancement, which may persist up to 8 months. Ring persistence on T1-weighted images should not be equated with treatment failure. Rather, T2-weighted images should be followed to see shrinkage of the necrotic center and capsular hypointensity.

Besides an obvious bacterial invasion through a traumatic or surgical event, pathogens may reach the brain by hematogenous seeding or direct extension from a contiguous focus. The brain is protected from infection by the calvaria, meninges, and physiologic blood-brain barrier. Once intracranial, bacteria may produce a severe inflammatory response due to the absence of lymphatics, lack of subarachnoid space capillaries, and the presence of Virchow-Robin spaces (perivascular CSF-containing spaces). Pathogenic bacteria may invade the brain itself, resulting in focal (abscess) or diffuse (encephalitis) lesions. The meninges may be affected (meningitis, ependymitis), as well as the epidural and subdural spaces (empyema). The most common focal infectious neurologic lesion is brain abscess. Most often, brain abscess is caused by hematogenous dissemination from an extracranial site, and the most common distant extracranial foci are pulmonary, then cardiac.[15] Septic thrombophlebitis involving emissary and cortical veins may result

in abscess formation adjacent to or distant from the primary focus. An abscess may also arise from an anatomically contiguous focus such as the middle ear, paranasal sinus, mastoid, or fascial space.[17] Intracranial spread of purulence from an oral focus involves movement of pus to the base of the skull along fascial planes. This route involves inoculation via fistulous tracts after osteitis of the adjacent bone and dural necrosis. Eventually, the cranium is violated by the venous route leading to sinus thrombosis or through the bone itself, causing leptomeningitis, subdural empyema, or brain abscess. Haymaker's[3] review of 28 fatal cases of neurologic infection after tooth extraction found brain abscess spread by the hematogenous route in 7 patients and 7 caused by direct inflammatory spread through the cranial bone itself. All cases were diagnosed at autopsy, and postmortem examination revealed several anatomic pathways: cellulitis extending from the extraction site along fascial planes to the base of the skull, along cranial nerve V_3 through the foramen ovale into the temporal lobe, through fracture of the maxillary sinus floor during maxillary extraction that led to cellulitis of the posterior orbit and frontal sinus, extension of sphenoid osteomyelitis, and submasseteric space infection extending into the infratemporal fossa and eventual temporal bone destruction. Once the brain is inoculated with a pathogen, a localized area of cerebritis forms. At this point, histologic examination reveals inflammatory cells, granulation tissue, and necrosis. Vascular congestion, edema, and petechial

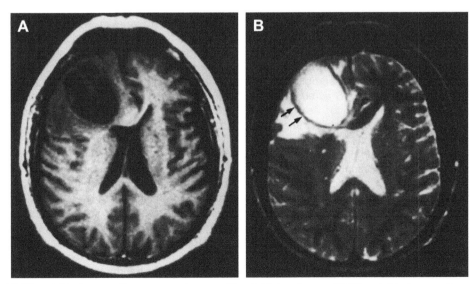

Fig. 6. (*A*) T1-weighted magnetic resonance image of frontal lobe abscess. (*B*) T2-weighted magnetic resonance image of the same frontal lobe abscess. (*From* Lazow SK, Kim D. Imaging head and neck infections. Oral and Maxillofac Surg Clin North Am 2001;13:587; with permission.)

hemorrhages are seen on gross examination. Eventually, over the space of a week, a capsule forms. As it thickens, the center becomes necrotic and liquefies. As the abscess matures, surrounding edema decreases. If the source of infection is the ear, chronic otitis media is the cause in more than 80% of cases. Acute otitis media usually leads to a subdural abscess. Otogenic brain abscesses are usually located in the temporal lobe or cerebellum and are rarely multiple. Sinusitis usually spreads to the frontal lobe. Facial infections, dural sinus thrombosis, and osteomyelitis result in frontal and temporal abscesses, and brain abscesses attributed to odontogenic foci most often occur in the temporal, parietal, and frontal lobes.

Bacterial findings in brain abscess mirror those of the primary focus. Acute infections are most often caused by aerobic organisms and chronic infections by anaerobes. Reporting of microbiological flora found in brain abscesses has varied. In the older literature, most brain abscesses attributed to dental infection have isolated a single organism, usually S viridans. However, brain abscesses are frequently polymicrobial.[18] Anaerobic and microaerophilic cocci and gram-negative and gram-positive anaerobic bacilli are the most often isolated organisms. Organisms most commonly associated with brain abscess in general are S aureus; aerobic, anaerobic, and microaerophilic streptococci, including α-hemolytic streptococci and Streptococcus milleri; Bacteroides; Enterobacteriaceae; and Pseudomonas. Less common causes are H influenzae, S pneumoniae, Neisseria meningitidis, Nocardia asteroides, Mycobacterium species, protozoa, fungi, helminths, and Treponema gondii. Specific organisms are seen with certain predisposing conditions. Penetrating trauma involves S aureus, aerobic streptococci, Enterobacteriaceae, and Clostridium. Congenital heart disease is associated with aerobic and microaerophilic streptococci and S aureus. Pulmonary infections, in addition to aerobic and anaerobic streptococci, may show anaerobic gram-negative bacilli (Prevotella, Porphyromonas, Bacteroides), Fusobacterium, Actinomyces, and Nocardia. Transplant recipients may manifest Aspergillus, Candida, Cryptococcus, Nocardia, and T gondii. HIV-positive patients also may involve T gondii, Mycobacterium, Cryptococcus, and Nocardia. Brain abscess caused by sinus and dental infections involves aerobic and anaerobic streptococci, anaerobic gram-negative bacilli, Fusobacterium, S aureus, and Enterobacteriaceae.[15] Most brain abscesses attributed to dental infection have had S viridans as the primary isolate. However, in a study of 60 brain abscesses,

Brewer and colleagues[19] found Streptococcus species in 32 of 60 cases, and S viridians in 18 of the 60 cases, yet attributed only 4 of the abscesses to odontogenic origin. Hollin and colleagues,[14] in a study of 5 brain abscesses, found 1 to be of odontogenic origin. However, this conclusion was based solely on the fact that the patient underwent multiple extractions over a several month period before development of a brain abscess, with a negative culture result (sterile abscess). Attributing a brain abscess to dental infection can only be confirmed by culture of identical strains of bacteria from the brain abscess and the oral infection. Corson and colleagues[1] report a case of odontogenic brain abscesses based on culture results of S milleri and Streptococcus sanguinis and the finding of several periodontally involved teeth. One of the teeth involved demonstrated a close association with the maxillary sinus. Mylonas and colleagues[20] report a case of cerebral abscess of odontogenic origin based on a concurrent finding of generalized periodontal disease, caries, and periapical pathology. In this case, the patient recovered after most of his teeth were extracted, and the brain abscess was resected. However, there is no mention of a culture result, and the investigators' literature search listed only 7 references relating cerebral abscess and dental infections. Often, case reports include the wordings possible, probable, and might in describing the causal relationship. Haymaker[3] studied 28 fatal neurologic infections after tooth extraction, concluding that the extraction initiated or precipitated the neurologic infection in all cases. Having the advantage of autopsy, the investigator found that 10 of the infections were spread by the hematogenous route and the other 18 by direct anatomic spread. The organism most frequently seen in the hematogenous spread group was Streptococcus and, in the direct spread group, Staphylococcus. However, only 1 of the 14 brain abscesses in the investigators' series had the same culture result as that of the oral focus, and that was S aureus.

Treatment of brain abscess commonly involves a combination of antibiotic therapy and surgery. If brain abscess is suspected, patients should be placed on antimicrobial therapy before surgical intervention. Current empirical regimens are tailored to the presumed source. Direct extension from sinuses, teeth, and middle ear is treated with penicillin G, metronidazole, and a third-generation cephalosporin. Hematogenous spread or penetrating trauma is treated with nafcillin, metronidazole, and a third-generation cephalosporin. Postoperative infections are treated with vancomycin (for methicillin-resistant S aureus) and ceftazidime or cefepime (for *Pseudomonas*). If no predisposing factor is apparent, vancomycin, metronidazole, and a third-generation cephalosporin should be administered. Surgery is the only way to precisely isolate the causative microorganism and tailor subsequent antibiotic therapy based on culture results. Traditionally 6 to 8 weeks of parenteral therapy is followed by 4 to 6 weeks of oral therapy. Surgical intervention is usually delayed until the surrounding capsule matures because mortality of patients undergoing treatment of the acute abscess is twice that of those with chronic abscess.[15] Only in rare cases are antibiotics the only form of therapy, which include multiple abscesses or an abscess in an inaccessible location, single abscess smaller than 2 cm, or a critically ill terminal patient. Surgical intervention may involve aspiration, incision and drainage, or excision. There has been an increasing tendency toward aspiration, although many studies show excision to be associated with more rapid resolution, decreased dosing time for antibiotic therapy, and a shorter hospital stay. Stereotactic techniques have greatly improved the precision of aspiration. Excision involves radical debulking of the lesion but not necessarily complete removal. Remnants may be left in areas of the motor cortex, internal capsule, and ventricular wall rather than risking hemiparesis or an open communication into the ventricular system. The mortality rate of brain abscess currently stands at 10%. However, if the abscess ruptures into the ventricular system, mortality increases to 80%.[15] The usefulness of HBO in the treatment of gas gangrene, refractory osteomyelitis, mycobacterial infections, and osteoradionecrosis has been well documented. There have been reports of HBO therapy being beneficial in isolated cases of aspergillosis, mucormycosis, coccidioidomycosis, and actinomycosis because reduction of tissue acidosis by increasing tissue perfusion resulted in a decrease in the growth rate of the fungal organism.

The prognosis of patients with brain abscess has improved markedly, primarily because of early diagnosis and treatment. Before the use of antibiotics, death was almost certain. Antibiotics and CT scanning have decreased the mortality rate to where it is today. The major prognostic indicator is the neurologic status of the patient at the time of diagnosis. The poorer the neurologic status on admission, the poorer is the long-range prognosis. Most obtunded or comatose patients do not survive. Excision followed by a course of appropriate antibiotic therapy is associated with the greatest chance for complete recovery without additional surgery. Persistent neurologic deficits depend on location and patient age. Children have a higher incidence of postoperative hemiparesis and seizures. Abscesses located in the parietal lobe are associated with more significant deficits than the frontal or temporal lobes. Also, hematogenous spread has been shown to result in more significant postinfection deficits than local invasion.

Brain abscess is a rare potentially life-threatening infection. Once almost certainly fatal, the mortality rate has dropped precipitously with the use of antibiotics and improved diagnostic tools such as CT. Reports of brain abscess as a result of dental infection have postulated that most of these infections reach the brain by CST or direct extension. However, both hematogenous and contiguous anatomic routes of spread are also suspected. Haymaker reported on 28 cases of neurologic spread of dental infection after tooth extraction, yet only 1 of 14 brain abscesses had the same bacteria cultured from both the brain and oral focus, and although 8 of the patients exhibited a dental focus (periodontoclasia, Vincent infection, oral sepsis), in the remaining 20 patients, the mouth was "clean." Corson and colleagues[1] reported a case of brain tumor caused by dental infection, with a dental focus (periodontitis) and a brain abscess culture result involving oral flora (*S milleri* and *S sanguinis*), yet point out that numerous cases attributed to dental infection have been reported in the literature even though the offending organism was not an oral pathogen (eg, *Escherichia coli*, *S aureus*). Yamamoto and colleagues[21] and Mueller and colleagues[22] have reported on brain abscesses caused by the *S milleri* group. In Mueller's series of 11 cases, 6 were thought to be of dental origin based on culture results. This finding far exceeds the incidence previously reported in other studies (<1%,[23] 2%,[24] 4%,[25] and 8.5%[26]). Although dental implication in development of brain abscess has historically been a diagnosis of exclusion, a thorough review of the literature reveals many abscesses with positive cultures with oral flora. However, there is rarely correlation with culture results from the supposed oral focus. With advanced technology such as DNA fingerprinting, it is possible to better pinpoint matching flora in the brain and oral cavity in the case of brain abscess and confirm what many already suspect: there is potential for spread of dental infection to neurologic structures, resulting in CST and brain abscess. Until evidence-based studies with matching bacterial serotypes and identical DNA homology, an obvious contiguous focus, and a documented pathway replace anecdotal reports, brain abscess secondary to dental infection will continue to be a diagnosis of exclusion.

REFERENCES

1. Corson MA, Postlethwaite KP, Seymour RA. Are dental infections a cause of brain abscess? Case report and review of the literature. Oral Dis 2001;7:61–5.
2. Flynn TR. Anatomy and surgery of deep fascial space infections of the head and neck. In: Kelly JP, editor, OMS knowledge update, vol. 1. Rosemont (IL): AAOMS; 1994. p. 104.
3. Haymaker W. Fatal infections of the central nervous system and meninges after tooth extraction with analysis of 28 cases. Am J Orthod Oral Surg 1945; 31:117–88.
4. Childs HG, Courville CB. Thrombosis of cavernous sinus secondary to dental infections. Am J Orthod Oral Surg 1942;28:367–515.
5. Rothwell P. Cerebrovascular diseases. In: Donaghy M, editor. Brain's diseases of the nervous system. 12th edition. Oxford (UK): Oxford University Press; 2009. p. 1084–6.
6. Mehrotra MC. Cavernous sinus thrombosis with generalized septicemia: report of a case following dental extraction. Oral Surg Oral Med Oral Pathol 1965;19:715–9.
7. Mazzeo V. Cavernous sinus thrombosis. J Oral Med 1974;29:53–6.
8. Taicher S, Garfunkel A, Feinsod M. Reversible cavernous sinus involvement due to minor dental infection: report of a case. Oral Surg Oral Med Oral Pathol 1978;46:7–9.
9. Yun MW, Hwang CF, Lui CC. Cavernous sinus thrombosis following odontogenic and cervicofacial infection. Eur Arch Otorhinolaryngol 1991;248:422–4.
10. Harbour RC, Trobe JD, Ballinger WE. Septic cavernous sinus thrombosis associated with gingivitis and parapharyngeal abscess. Arch Ophthalmol 1984;102:94–7.
11. Feldman DP, Picerno NA, Porubsky ES. Cavernous sinus thrombosis complicating odontogenic parapharyngeal space neck abscess: a case report and discussion. Otolaryngol Head Neck Surg 2000;123:744–5.
12. Colbert S, Cameron M, Williams J. Septic thrombosis of the cavernous sinus and dental infection. Br J Oral Maxillofac Surg 2010;48:1–2.
13. Ogundiya DA, Keith DA, Mirowski J. Cavernous sinus thrombosis and blindness as complications of an odontogenic infection. J Oral Maxillofac Surg 1989;47:1317–21.
14. Hollin SA, Hayashi H, Gross SW. Intracranial abscesses of odontogenic origin. Oral Surg Oral Med Oral Pathol 1967;23:277–9.
15. Nath A. Brain abscess and parameningeal infections. In: Goldman L, Ausiello D, editors. Cecil medicine. 23rd edition. Philadelphia: Saunders Elsevier; 2007. p. 2771–6. Chapter 438.
16. Britt RH, Enzmann DR. Clinical stages of human brain abscesses on serial CT scans after contrast infusion: computerized tomographic, neuropathological, and clinical correlations. J Neurosurg 1983; 59:972–89.
17. Mampalam T, Rosenblum M. Trends in the management of bacterial brain abscesses: a review of 102 cases over 17 years. Neurosurgery 1988; 23:451–7.
18. Brook I. Aerobic and anaerobic bacteriology of intracranial abscesses. Pediatr Neurol 1992;8:210–4.
19. Brewer MS, MacCarty CS, Wellman WE. Brain abscess: a review of recent experience. Ann Intern Med 1975;82:571–6.
20. Mylonas AI, Tzerbos FH, Mihalaki M, et al. Cerebral abscess of odontogenic origin. J Craniomaxillofac Surg 2007;35:63–7.
21. Yamamoto M, Fukushima T, Ohshiro S, et al. Brain abscess caused by Streptococcus intermedius: two case reports. Surg Neurol 1999;51:219–22.
22. Mueller AA, Saldamli B, Stubinger S, et al. Oral bacterial cultures in nontraumatic brain abscesses: results of a first-line study. Oral Surg Oral Med Oral Pathol Oral Radiol Endod 2009;107:469–76.
23. Roche M, Humphreys H, Smyth E, et al. A twelve-year review of central nervous system bacterial abscesses; presentation and aetiology. Clin Microbiol Infect 2003;9:803–9.
24. Sichizya K, Fieggen G, Taylor A, et al. Brain abscesses—the Groote Schuur experience. 1993-2003. S Afr J Surg 2005;43:79–82.
25. Carpenter J, Stapleton S, Holliman R. Retrospective analysis of 49 cases of brain abscess and review of the literature. Eur J Clin Microbiol Infect Dis 2007;26: 1–11.
26. Prasad KN, Mishra AM, Gupta D, et al. Analysis of microbiological etiology and mortality in patients with brain abscess. J Infect 2006;53:221–7.

How Do We Manage Oral Infections in Allogeneic Stem Cell Transplantation and Other Severely Immunocompromised Patients?

Stefan Palmason, DMD[a,b],*, Francisco M. Marty, MD[c],
Nathaniel S. Treister, DMD, DMSc[a,b]

KEYWORDS

- Immunocompromise • Neutropenia • Infection
- Odontogenic • Oral

Since its introduction in the 1950s, enormous progress has been made in the field of hematopoietic cell transplantation (HCT), where it now has become the standard treatment for many hematologic malignancies and bone marrow failure syndromes.[1,2] The use of intensive conditioning regimens with the resulting depletion of cell-mediated immunity and loss of mucosal integrity greatly increases the risk of localized and systemic infections in this patient population.[3,4] Classically, it takes patients 10 to 35 days to recover from the profound pancytopenia after stem cell infusion, depending on the stem cell source. In addition, immune reconstitution after HCT is a prolonged process, and long-term immunosuppressive therapies are often necessary to prevent or manage graft-versus-host disease (GVHD) in recipients of allogeneic grafts.[5,6] Although the increased use of reduced intensity conditioning regimens for allogeneic HCT has led to a decreased risk of infection and mortality in the early posttransplant period, these patients often require long-term immunosuppressive therapy.[7] Despite significant advances in the prevention and management of infectious diseases in HCT recipients, infections remain a primary cause of morbidity and mortality.[8–12]

The oral cavity is among the most susceptible sites for infection in the human body. With normal immune function, adequate salivary flow, and appropriate preventive measures, the oral cavity can generally be kept free of infectious diseases. Oral infections in the immunocompetent population are largely of odontogenic origin, with fungal and viral infections occurring far less frequently. In severely immunocompromised patients, such as those undergoing allogeneic HCT, risk of infection is not only significantly increased, but infections in these patients may present with unusual patterns, resolve slowly despite prolonged and intensive therapy, and in some cases become

The authors have no relevant conflict of interests to disclose.

a Division of Oral Medicine and Dentistry, Brigham and Women's Hospital, 1620 Tremont Street, Boston, MA 02120, USA

b Department of Oral Medicine, Infection and Immunity, Harvard School of Dental Medicine, 188 Longwood Avenue, Boston, MA 02115, USA

c Division of Infectious Diseases, Brigham and Women's Hospital, Dana-Farber Cancer Institute, Harvard Medical School, 75 Francis Street, Boston, MA 02115, USA

* Corresponding author.

E-mail address: spalmason@partners.org

Oral Maxillofacial Surg Clin N Am 23 (2011) 579–599
doi:10.1016/j.coms.2011.07.012

life-threatening.[13] Localized oral infections caused by a variety of bacterial, fungal, and viral species may result in disseminated disease because of prolonged neutropenia, especially in the context of mucositis and breach of the protective mucosal barrier.[3,14–16]

This article reviews the most frequently encountered oral infections in patients undergoing allogeneic HCT with respect to clinical presentation, prevention, diagnosis, and management. Although the primary focus of this article is on patients undergoing allogeneic HCT, the following descriptions of manifestations and principles of diagnosis and management can be extended to other similarly immunocompromised patients, such as recipients of solid organ transplants, AIDS patients, and patients with autoimmune and other immune-mediated diseases undergoing long-term intensive immunosuppressive therapy.

VIRAL INFECTIONS
Herpes Simplex Virus

Herpes simplex virus (HSV) infections are among the most prevalent infectious diseases affecting humans.[17] HSV-1 primarily infects the orofacial area and HSV-2 primarily causes genital infections, although occasionally this can be reversed.[18–20] Data from the US National Health and Nutritional Examination Survey (1999–2004) demonstrated an overall seroprevalence in persons age 19 to 49 of 57.7% for HSV-1 and 17% for HSV-2, with higher figures in older individuals and those from lower socioeconomic groups.[21]

Most primary HSV-1 infections are asymptomatic and occur during childhood, although there has been an increasing incidence reported in young adults.[22,23] When clinical disease develops, signs and symptoms include erythema and ulceration of the intraoral keratinized and nonkeratinized mucosa (eg, gingivostomatitis), lymphadenopathy, fever, malaise, and pain.[22] After primary infection, HSV-1 establishes latency, usually in the trigeminal ganglion.[24] Recrudescent orofacial HSV-1 lesions occur in 20% to 40% of the healthy population with most cases presenting periorally as recurrent herpes labialis and only rarely as intraoral ulcerations that are restricted to the keratinized tissues.[25,26] Factors associated with viral reactivation include stress, sun exposure, and illness; however, asymptomatic viral shedding (during which transmission is possible) is more than two times more frequent than recrudescent outbreaks.[25,27]

Recrudescent oral HSV infection is common in the severely immunocompromised patient and may develop despite antiviral prophylaxis. Cell-mediated immunity, which is significantly depressed following HCT, plays the principal role in controlling HSV infections.[28] Compared with immunocompetent individuals, oral HSV infections in immunocompromised patients are typically larger and more extensive, frequently affect intraoral keratinized and nonkeratinized tissues, and have a more aggressive and painful course that is not self-limiting and requires therapy (**Fig. 1**).[29–31] HSV infection can result in disseminated and sometimes life-threatening infections including fulminant hepatitis, pneumonitis, and encephalitis.[14,32–35] In all severely immunocompromised patients who present with acute onset of painful oral ulcerations, HSV infection must be considered.

Other Relevant Herpes Species

There are several other viruses of the herpes family that are of relevance in the oral cavity. Although oral conditions caused by these viruses are encountered much less frequently than HSV infections, it is essential for the clinician to know their signs and symptoms. Oral manifestations in association with human herpes virus (HHV)-6 and -7 have rarely been reported and therefore are not discussed further.

Varicella zoster virus

Varicella zoster virus (VZV) reactivations previously occurred in approximately 30% of HCT recipients in the first year post-transplantation but this has been reduced to less than 5% with antiviral prophylaxis.[36,37] Reactivation of VZV inside the oral cavity is very rare; 1.7% of all VZV reactivations involve the V2 or V3 branches of the trigeminal nerve.[38]

Several days of prodromal pain is common, followed by unilateral blisters that erupt to form ulcers on the skin. Lesions typically affect the thoracic or lumbar dermatomes but the trigeminal nerve can be involved in 11.8% of cases, with most involving the ophthalmic branch.[38] In severely immunocompromised patients, multiple bilateral sites can be involved and these infections can potentially lead to life-threatening disseminated visceral infections (eg, encephalitis, pneumonitis, myocarditis, and hepatitis; **Fig. 2**).[39,40] Intraoral lesions are still rare and are largely restricted to the keratinized mucosa, appearing similar to those of HSV. Alveolar bone necrosis with tooth exfoliation is a rare but reported complication.[41] Peripheral facial palsy can also occur in association with VZV reactivation.[42] Zoster sine herpete is a presentation of pain symptoms without involvement of the dermatomes and can present with facial palsy.[43,44] Postherpetic

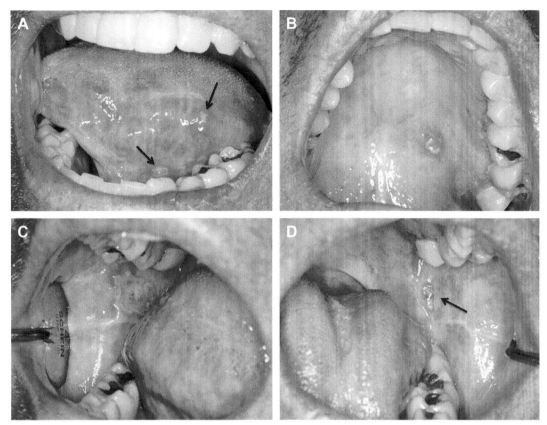

Fig. 1. Extensive HSV recrudescence in a 45 year-old male 7 months status-post allogeneic hematopoietic cell transplantation from a mismatched unrelated donor for chronic lymphocytic leukemia. Ulcerations of the (*A*) left lateral tongue (*arrows*); (*B*) left hard palate, with focal ulceration toward the midline and croplike ulcerations along the gingival margin extending from the premolars to the tuberosity; (*C*) right buccal mucosa; and (*D*) left buccal mucosa (*arrow*).

neuralgia (PHN) has been reported to affect 35% of HCT patients with herpes zoster reactivation, which is higher than the 9% incidence in the immunocompetent population.[45] Antiviral therapy after reactivation may help reduce the risk of developing PHN.[46] The zoster vaccine (Zostavax, Merck, Whitehouse Station, NJ) has been found to reduce the burden of illness of herpes zoster and incidence of PHN by more than 60% in non-immunocompromised hosts.[47] Because it is a live-attenuated vaccine, it is not currently recommended for HCT recipients early after transplant, but could be considered in patients who are 2 years post-HCT and on no immunosuppression.

Epstein-Barr Virus

Epstein-Barr virus (EBV) infections are usually contracted through saliva and can cause infectious mononucleosis, lymphoproliferative disorders, nasopharyngeal carcinoma, and oral hairy leukoplakia. The only one of these conditions that is

encountered with an increased frequency in the allogeneic HCT patient population is post-transplant lymphoproliferative disorder (PTLD).

PTLD typically presents during the first year post-HCT with most cases associated with EBV-infected transformed B cells that present with extranodal disease.[48–51] Recently, a trend toward increased PTLD has been noticed in patients receiving either umbilical cord blood transplants (because of the absence of antigen-experienced mature T cells) or reduced-intensity conditioning regimens (likely resulting from inadequate B-cell depletion).[52] Without treatment, mortality is very high, but with current management strategies survival approaches 90%.[53] Seronegative HCT recipients (10% of adult population) are at risk to contract EBV from their donor and seroconversion as high as 95% has been reported.[54–56] PTLD is therefore more frequent in children because primary infections contracted near to the time of HCT are more likely to cause PTLD than recurrent infections.[57,58] In addition, profound T-cell

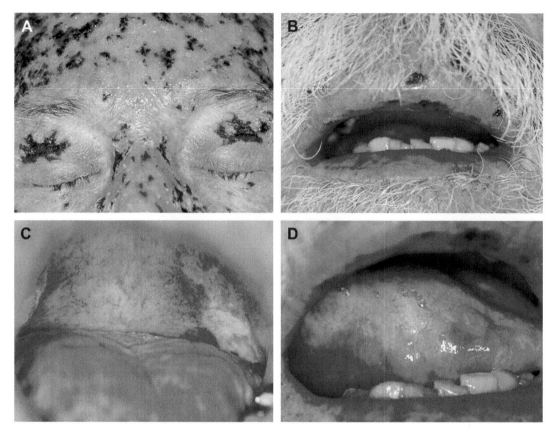

Fig. 2. Disseminated VZV in a 57 year-old male day +78 status-post allogeneic hematopoietic stem cell transplantation from an unrelated donor for acute myelogenous leukemia. Hemorrhagic crusts of the (*A*) skin, (*B*) upper lip, (*C*) soft palate, and (*D*) right lateral tongue.

immunosuppression is a risk factor because it results in a lack of suppression of B-cell proliferation.[59] Gastrointestinal involvement is seen in two-thirds of cases, and in approximately one-quarter of cases the head and neck area is involved.[50,60,61] One recent study speculates that the use of molecular EBV monitoring has shifted the presentation of PTLD to a milder phenotype because of earlier detection.[62]

Oral PTLD lesions present as mucosal swellings, nonhealing ulcers, or intraosseous radiolucent lesions (**Fig. 3**).[60] As is the case in other parts of the body, biopsy is necessary to confirm the diagnosis.[50] Treatment options include reduction of immunosuppression, rituximab, and other chemotherapy regimens.[59]

Cytomegalovirus

The age-adjusted seroprevalence of cytomegalovirus (CMV) infection is 50%, and it is one of the most frequent causes of infection after HCT; however, CMV only rarely presents with oral cavity lesions.[63,64] Primary infection is often asymptomatic, and although the mechanism of

latency is not clear, the salivary glands, endothelial tissue, neutrophils, and dendritic cells have all been found to contain the virus.[65] Reactivation in immunocompromised patients can lead to

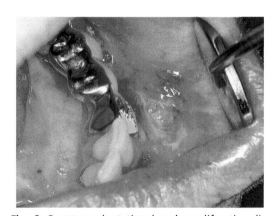

Fig. 3. Post-transplantation lymphoproliferative disease that presented as a focal ulceration of the left buccal vestibule in a 56 year-old female who was day +60 status-post reduced-intensity post–reduced-intensity double umbilical cord blood allogeneic hematopoietic cell transplantation.

pneumonitis, colitis and enteritis, retinitis, hepatitis, and other organ involvement.[66,67] CMV monitoring is performed through quantitative CMV antigenemia or quantitative CMV polymerase chain reaction.[68]

Oral lesions secondary to CMV reactivation are characterized by painful nonspecific ulceration that is typically solitary, although multiple ulcerations can occur. These can clinically mimic major aphthous ulcers. Biopsy is required for diagnosis because the virus and cellular changes are typically only seen deep in the endothelium of the connective tissue.[69]

Human Herpes Virus 8

HHV-8 is a herpes virus of the gamma family, related to EBV.[70] Although HHV-8 infection is frequent in endemic countries in the Mediterranean, Middle East, and Africa, where the seroprevalence is as high as 50%, the seroprevalence in healthy United States blood donors is only 7.3%.[71]

HHV-8 is known as a causative agent in Kaposi sarcoma, which frequently presents with intraoral lesions.[72] Kaposi sarcoma has been documented to occur in patients receiving immunosuppressive therapy but is most frequently seen in HIV-infected patients.[73,74] Kaposi sarcoma has only rarely been reported after HCT, although a recent report described oral Kaposi sarcoma erupting in an HHV-8 seronegative patient almost 5 years post allogeneic HCT.[70,75] Although initial clinical presentation is usually a flat lesion ranging from red to purple in color, the later stages are characterized by masses that can become large and ulcerated (**Fig. 4**).[76]

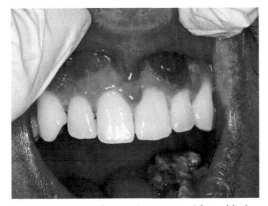

Fig. 4. Disseminated Kaposi sarcoma with oral lesions of the maxillary buccal gingiva and the left retromolar pad in a 64 year-old HIV+ male with a CD4+ count of 30 cells/mm³ who was not compliant with his antiretroviral therapy regimen.

Other Relevant Viruses

Human Papillomaviruses

Of more than 100 types of human papillomaviruses (HPV) that have been identified in the oral cavity and oropharynx there are 25 that have been found in oral lesions.[77] Although HPV 6 and 11 are most frequently found in benign lesions, HPV 16 and 18 have been linked to the development of oropharyngeal cancer.[78,79] Four presentations of HPV-related oral lesions have been characterized: squamous papilloma, verruca vulgaris, condyloma accuminatum, and focal epithelial hyperplasia, with squamous papillomas being found to occur in 1 in 250 healthy adults.[80] Occurrence of HPV-associated oral benign or malignant lesions post-HCT has not been reported in the literature.

Enteroviruses

Although not reported in the HCT setting, enteroviral infections, such as herpangina and hand-foot-and-mouth disease, should be considered in the differential diagnosis when multiple aphthous-like lesions occur in association with influenza-like symptoms with an acute onset.[81]

FUNGAL INFECTIONS
Candidiasis

The most common fungal infection in the oral cavity of humans is caused by *Candida albicans*, a yeast that has been found to be commensal in nearly 20% of the normal population, whereas the incidence of all yeasts is 35%.[82] Other frequent candidal species include *C tropicalis* and *C glabrata* and together these three comprise more than 80% of specimens isolated from the oral cavity.[82,83] Recent data suggest that up to 11% of yeast isolates from denture wearers can include *C dubliniensis*, which has been identified as an emerging opportunistic pathogen in immunocompromised individuals.[83–86] In one study of patients with hematologic malignancies undergoing HCT or chemotherapy, 65% of isolates from the oral cavity consisted of *C albicans*.[87] Other species isolated from immunocompromised patients include *C krusei*, *C tropicalis*, *C glabrata*, *C parapsilosis*, *C cerevisiae*, *C famata*, and *C dubliniensis*.[85,87,88]

Several local or systemic factors have been identified that predispose individuals to developing oropharyngeal fungal infection, including reduced salivary flow and function, use of prostheses, decreased immune status, use of intraoral topical steroids, and imbalance in the oral microflora often caused by the use of antibiotics.[82] The immune system has a variety of mechanisms that are important in the control and prevention of oropharyngeal candidiasis. Granulocytes, such as neutrophils, play a primary role by phagocytosing yeast organisms.[89] Cell-mediated immunity also plays an important role, with cytokine production (eg, interferon-gamma) by T cells enhancing leukocyte microbicidal activity.[90] Humoral immunity is also important because salivary IgA reduces the epithelial adherence of *C albicans*.[91] Patients undergoing myeloablative HCT are at high risk for developing fungal infections during the neutropenic period and are placed on antifungal prophylaxis at many centers. Patients undergoing allogeneic transplantation may remain at high risk for developing infection because of delayed immune reconstitution and immunosuppression secondary to prophylaxis and management of GVHD.

Pseudomembranous candidiasis is the most frequently encountered presentation in the oral cavity (**Fig. 5**A). It presents as symptomatic or asymptomatic white curd-like plaques that can typically be easily wiped off with a tongue blade or gauze, revealing an erythematous base. *Candida* species do not typically penetrate the keratin layer and the presence of ulcers should therefore raise suspicion of a different etiology. Erythematous candidiasis presents as an erythematous patch on the dorsal aspect of the tongue, palate (following the outline of the denture in those wearing dentures), or buccal mucosa; however, this diagnosis should always be suspected in susceptible patients who report oral burning symptoms, even when there is minimal evidence of mucosal erythema, because findings may be subtle (see **Fig. 5**B). It has most frequently

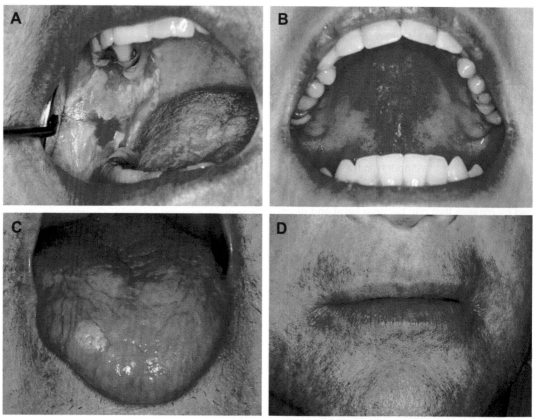

Fig. 5. Oral candidiasis clinical presentations. (*A*) Pseudomembranous candidiasis of the right buccal mucosa that developed secondary to topical clobetasol therapy for management of an intraoral systemic lupus erythematosus lesion in a 30 year-old female. (*B*) Fluconazole-resistant erythematous candidiasis of the palate secondary to combined topical clobetasol and tacrolimus therapy in a 57 year-old female who was 16 months status-post allogeneic hematopoietic cell transplantation for acute myelogenous leukemia. (*C*) Hyperplastic candidiasis of the right tongue dorsum in the setting of long-term topical corticosteroid therapy for oral chronic GVHD in a 64 year-old male 8 years status-post allogeneic hematopoietic cell transplantation. (*D*) Angular cheilitis in the setting of salivary gland hypofunction in a 48 year-old male status-post allogeneic therapy for non-Hodgkin lymphoma of the nasal cavity.

been associated with salivary gland hypofunction, denture wearing, corticosteroids, and broad-spectrum antibacterials.[92] Hyperplastic candidiasis is a rare manifestation characterized by a well-defined slightly raised white lesion that cannot be rubbed away and appears clinically as leukoplakia; therefore, biopsy is necessary to rule out premalignant changes (see **Fig. 5**C). Angular cheilitis presents as fissures and erythema in the corners of the mouth and is often associated with concurrent intraoral infection (see **Fig. 5**D). These lesions can also be coinfected with *Staphylococcus aureus*.

Invasive Fungal Infections

Invasive fungal infections in patients undergoing HCT can be broadly divided into invasive candidiasis (25% of cases) and invasive mold infections (75% of cases).[93] The incidence of invasive candidiasis in patients undergoing allogeneic HCT has been reported to be 4.6% and is associated with a mortality rate of 20%; the most frequent species are *C glabrata* followed by *C parapsilosis* and *C krusei*.[94] It has been suggested that candidemia and infection of internal organs is often preceded by oropharyngeal candidiasis.[95,96]

Generally of much greater concern are noncandidal invasive fungal infections caused by molds that typically infect the respiratory tract (lungs or sinuses) and can present intraorally as yellow, grey, or black pseudomembranous ulceration with a necrotic base.[97,98] Invasive fungal infections affecting the oral cavity most frequently arise from direct extension from the maxillary sinus (typically presenting as an erosion of the hard palate or posterior tongue), but can also develop because of direct inoculation or hematogenous dissemination.[97,98] Aspergillosis is a relatively common opportunistic fungal infection of the orofacial area in patients receiving chemotherapy for hematologic malignancies, with an incidence of 10% or higher.[92,98–102] Other invasive fungal infections that can present with oral involvement include histoplasmosis and zygomycosis, with over half of all cases affecting craniofacial structures.[92,103]

Gooley and colleagues[9] compared the frequency of invasive fungal infections in HCT patients between the periods of 1993 to 1997 and 2003 to 2007 and found an 88% reduction in invasive candidal infections, and a 51% reduction in invasive mold infections in the later period. Furthermore, 12-week mortality rates in HCT recipients with aspergillosis have been markedly reduced from the 1990s (reported as high as 80%) and recently have been reported to be 35%.[101] This is largely attributable to the introduction of new wide-spectrum antifungal agents, improved monitoring, and the widespread use of reduced-intensity conditioning regimens.[9]

BACTERIAL INFECTIONS
Bacteremia

Bacteremia is a potentially fatal complication in severely immunocompromised patients. Organisms that may potentially arise from the oral cavity and have been isolated from blood cultures in patients undergoing allogeneic HCT include *Streptococcal* sp (eg, *S mitis*), *Leptotrichia buccalis*, *Fusobacterium nucleatum*, and *S aureus*. Poor dental health has been associated with an increased risk of streptococcal bacteremias during post-HCT neutropenic periods.[104] One longitudinal study of more than 40,000 patients with cancer and febrile neutropenia demonstrated an overall mortality rate less than 10%; however, those with gram-positive or gram-negative bacteremias had mortality rates of 21% and 34%, respectively.[105] As a consequence of systemic antibacterial prophylaxis directed against gram-negative enteric organisms, there has been a shift toward an increased proportion of gram-positive bacteremias.[106]

Odontogenic Infections

Most bacterial infections in the oral cavity originate from teeth or their surrounding structures. These infections are broadly divided into periapical infections that originate from nonvital teeth, and periodontal infections that originate from the supporting structures of teeth. Acute infections are usually managed before HCT but chronic periapical and periodontal infections can easily be neglected because of their often indolent and asymptomatic courses. These chronic infections can progress and become acute, resulting in odontogenic abscesses, in particular in the context of immunosuppression. In the severely immunosuppressed patient odontogenic infections can have an atypical presentation without the usual clinical features of erythema, swelling, and purulence.

Endodontic Infections

Periapical infections are polymicrobial with a combination of facultative and strict anaerobes, the latter of which tend to predominate.[107] Although facultative anaerobes include viridans streptococci and *Enterococcus faecalis*, most strict anaerobes consist of *Bacteroides forsythus*.[108–110] Additional species include the anginosus group streptococci, *Porphyromonas*, *Prevotella*, *Peptostreptococcus*, and *Fusobacterium*.[107]

Periapical infections can erode through the alveolar bone and tend to follow the path of least resistance when spreading into soft tissue spaces.[111] Most periapical infections extend buccally within the space defined by the attachments of the buccinator muscle, resulting in intraoral abscess formation.[112] Infection arising from mandibular molars may spread lingually, leading to infection in the submandibular spaces. Maxillary periapical infections can potentially spread to the nasal cavity or the maxillary sinuses resulting in sinusitis characterized by pain, headaches, and maxillary tenderness.[111,113] More severe complications of periapical infections, including Ludwig angina and cavernous sinus thrombosis, are not encountered at any greater frequency in HCT patients. However, in profoundly neutropenic patients, infections may lead to localized areas of hard and soft tissue necrosis that can be very painful and generally only resolve with cell count recovery (**Fig. 6**).

Periodontal Infections

Periodontal organisms in normal hosts consist mainly of *Streptococcus* sp, *Actinomyces* sp, *Peptostreptococcus*, *F nucleatum*, *Porphyromonas gingivalis*, and *Prevotella intermedia*. In immunocompromised hosts, increases in *Klebsiella pneumoniae*, *Pseudomonas* species, *C albicans*, staphylococci, and enteric bacilli have been reported.[114] Periodontal disease is generally chronic; however, the condition may be acutely exacerbated during prolonged periods of neutropenia resulting in acute periodontal infection. There is evidence that suggests that poor periodontal health is associated with increased bacteremia in patients receiving high-dose chemotherapy.[114] Locally, severe necrotizing ulcerative gingivitis or periodontitis is characterized by painful necrotic ulceration that can extend to adjacent tissues

(eg, palatal mucosa) and can develop acutely in patients with advanced periodontal disease (**Fig. 7**).[115–117]

Pericoronitis can arise from partially erupted third molars even in the healthy population.[118] Although this can result in painful swelling with soft tissue ulceration and necrosis, a recent study found no increase in systemic infections in HCT patients with pericoronitis (**Fig. 8**).[119]

Nonodontogenic Infections

Nonodontogenic oral bacterial infections are very rare, but can present as localized soft tissue abscesses arising secondary to soft tissue trauma (eg, bite injury) or as necrotizing stomatitis, which is clinically similar to acute necrotizing periodontitis but without an obvious odontogenic etiology. Tonsillar and salivary gland infections have not been reported to occur at an increased frequency in this patient population.

PREVENTION
Pre-HCT Dental Treatment

When feasible, the most effective approach to management of oral infections is prevention. With respect to odontogenic infections and risk of bacteremia in patients undergoing HCT, all potential oral sources of infection should be eliminated before the initiation of conditioning therapy. This requires a comprehensive pre-HCT oral evaluation that can efficiently and conveniently be completed off-site by a patient's local dentist who is guided by detailed written instructions from the oncology service.[120] Treatment ideally should be completed at least 2 weeks before admission for HCT.[121]

The oral evaluation should include a history of any symptomatic teeth, comprehensive extraoral and intraoral examination, and radiographic evaluation including a full mouth series and a panoramic

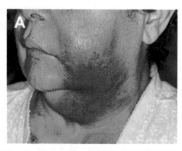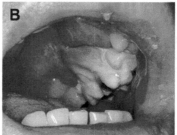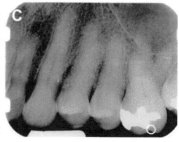

Fig. 6. Atypical presentation of an endodontic lesion in a 65 year-old female with prolonged severe neutropenia after reinduction chemotherapy for relapsed pre–B cell acute lymphoblastic leukemia 2 years status-post allogeneic hematopoietic cell transplantation. (*A*) Firm erythematous facial swelling in the left buccal region extending to the left submandibular area. (*B*) Area of hard and soft tissue necrosis of the palate. (*C*) Periapical radiograph demonstrating a very small periapical radiolucency associated with tooth #14.

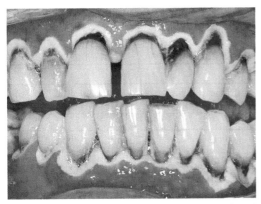

Fig. 7. Marginal gingival necrosis in a 59 year-old female with pre-exisiting periodontal disease who was undergoing induction chemotherapy for acute myelogenous leukemia and was profoundly neutropenic.

film.[122] All caries should be eliminated and defective restorations replaced. Heavily restored teeth should be assessed for vitality, and nonvital teeth should be treated with endodontic therapy or extraction. Persistent periapical radiolucencies in previously endodontically treated teeth that are asymptomatic do not seem to be associated with an increased risk of infectious complications and therefore do not require retreatment or extraction.[123] Symptomatic impacted third molars should be considered for extraction to minimize any potential infection risk.[121] Scaling and prophylaxis should be completed, and any teeth with advanced periodontal bone loss and mobility should be extracted.[124] Before any invasive dental procedures, the complete blood cell count should be reviewed with particular attention to the platelet count and absolute neutrophil count. There is no evidence that patients require

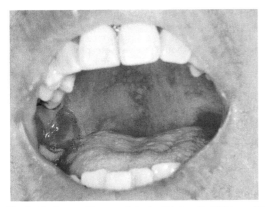

Fig. 8. Pericoronitis associated with tooth #32 in a 40 year-old male receiving reinduction chemotherapy for acute myelogenous leukemia.

antibiotic prophylaxis before delivery of dental care; however, a therapeutic course of antibiotics should be considered in patients who are neutropenic. Patients who are thrombocytopenic (in particular with a platelet count <20,000 cells/μL) may require a platelet transfusion before invasive procedures if excessive bleeding is expected.

Oral Hygiene Regimens

Chlorhexidine gluconate (swish and spit), nystatin (swish and swallow), and clotrimazole troches are frequently used for oral antimicrobial decontamination in HCT patients. Chlorhexidine is an effective antibacterial agent with antifungal activity; alcohol-free formulations may be better tolerated especially in the context of mucositis.[125] The use of soft toothbrushes has not been found to increase gram-positive bacteremia[125]; however, some centers prefer to use sponge brushes to reduce the risk of gingival bleeding caused by thrombocytopenia. The 2009 guidelines from the American Society for Blood and Marrow Transplantation recommend brushing with a soft toothbrush two to three times a day and flossing gently once a day, as tolerated, even during periods of neutropenia.[126]

Oral appliances must be kept clean. Dentures should be brushed gently and disinfected for 20 to 30 minutes daily with nystatin, chlorhexidine, or 1:10 diluted sodium hypochlorite. Dentures should be kept out of the mouth during the night and are generally not tolerated if mucositis is present.

Systemic Prophylactic Agents

In 2009 the American Society for Blood and Marrow Transplantation reported thorough guidelines on the prevention of infectious complications in HCT recipients (**Table 1**).[126]

Acyclovir (Zovirax) prophylaxis is provided for all seropositive patients to prevent recrudescent HSV infections. Antiviral prophylaxis with acyclovir has been demonstrated to reduce the rate of reactivation from 70% to less than 5%.[31,127–130] Oral valacyclovir (Valtrex) has been found to be as effective as oral and intravenous acyclovir in neutropenic patients.[131,132] Low-dose acyclovir is effective against HSV and VZV. High-dose acyclovir or ganciclovir (Cytovene) are sometimes used for CMV prophylaxis.

Fluconazole (Diflucan) is frequently used for prevention of invasive candidiasis and at some centers is started at the initiation of conditioning and continued at least through the neutropenic period.[133,134] Prolonged fluconazole prophylaxis for at least 75 days post-transplantation has been

Table 1
ASBMT guidelines for antimicrobial prophylactic regimens in HCT patients

First Line			Alternative	
Antibacterial agents[a]				
Levofloxacin	500 mg p.o. QD		Azithromycin	250 mg QD
Ciprofloxacin	500 mg p.o. BID			
Antiviral agents				
HSV[b]	Acyclovir	400–800 mg p.o. BID 250 mg/m^2/dose i.v. every 12 h	Valacyclovir	500 mg p.o. BID
VZV[c]	VZV Ig (postexposure)	5 vials (125 units each)	Valacyclovir[d]	1 g p.o. TID
	Acyclovir (reactivation)	800 mg p.o. BID for 1 y	Valacyclovir	500 mg p.o. BID for 1 y
CMV[e]	Ganciclovir (prophylaxis)	5 mg/kg/dose i.v. BID for 5–7 d then QD until Day +100	Foscarnet	60 mg/kg i.v. BID for 7 d then 90–120 mg/kg QD until Day +100
			Acyclovir	500 mg/m^2 i.v. TID 800 mg p.o QID
			Valacyclovir	2 g p.o. TID-QID
	Monitoring CMV-DNA polymerase chain reaction CMV pp65 antigenemia Preemptive treatment Ganciclovir	5 mg/kg/dose i.v. BID for 7–14 d then QD until indicator test is negative	Foscarnet (cidofovir or valganciclovir can be used if necessary)	60 mg/kg i.v. BID for 7–14 d then 90 mg/kg QD until indicator test is negative
Antifungal agents[f]				
Fluconazole	400 mg p.o. QD 400 mg i.v. QD		Fluconazole	200 mg p.o./i.v. QD
			Itraconazole	200 mg oral solution BID
			Micafungin	50 mg i.v. QD
			Voriconazole	4 mg/kg i.v. BID or 200 mg p.o. BID
			Posaconazole	200 mg p.o. TID

[a] Adults anticipated to be neutropenic for 7 days or more, started at Day 0 and continued until recover from neutropenia.
[b] Starting from the beginning of conditioning therapy and continued until engraftment or until mucositis resolves.
[c] If exposed to varicella or zoster then postexposure prophylaxis should be initiated if the patient is not more than 2 years out of transplant or if he is on immunosuppressive therapy or has chronic GVHD. If a patient receiving conditioning therapy is exposed to a vaccinee that has developed signs of primary disease he should receive postexposure prophylaxis. If the patient has signs or symptoms of reactivation then initiate prophylaxis of disease reactivation.
[d] Day 3–22 after exposure.
[e] Prophylaxis or preemptive strategies can be used. In preemptive strategy treatment is initiated if monitoring tests are positive for CMV. These strategies can be combined in seropositive patients receiving cord blood transplant. Prophylaxis strategy is generally used in seronegative recipients independent of donor status. In addition to this those at increased risk for CMV disease undergo preemptive strategy until immunocompetent but that is beyond the scope of this article.
[f] From the start of conditioning until engraftment.
Adapted from Tomblyn M, Chiller T, Einsele H, et al. Guidelines for preventing infectious complications among hematopoietic cell transplant recipients: a global perspective. Bone Marrow Transplant 2009;44(8):453–558; with permission.

associated with decreased candidiasis-related mortality in one transplant center.[135] It should be kept in mind that *C krusei* is resistant and *C glabrata* can become resistant to fluconazole; documented infection with either generally requires broader-spectrum azole antifungal therapy or treatment with a different class of antifungal medication.[136] Posaconazole (Noxafil) is approved for invasive fungal infection prophylaxis in some immunocompromised patients and may be more beneficial than fluconazole and itraconazole (Sporanox) in neutropenic patients.[137] Micafungin (Mycamine) is the only echinocandin that has been approved for antifungal prophylaxis in HCT.[138] The use of both posaconazole and micafungin remains limited because of cost and the need for intravenous administration.

Systemic antibacterial prophylaxis with a fluoroquinolone (levofloxacin [Levaquin]) has been recommended to prevent bloodstream infections in patients who are expected to be neutropenic for 7 or more days, especially when being treated on an outpatient basis.[139,140] Quinolones are used because of their broad-spectrum activity and the lack of myelosuppression; however, there is increasing prevalence of quinolone-resistant gram-negative bacteria and staphylococcal species.[126,141] There are no indications for routine prophylaxis against gram-positive bacteria. With respect to the oral flora, penicillin and quinolone resistance in viridans streptococci has been reported.[142,143] There is no consensus on the use of growth factor therapy to reduce the period of neutropenia because this has not been demonstrated to reduce the rate of infection.[126]

MANAGEMENT
Noninfectious Oral Lesions

It is critical for the clinician to be able to recognize the characteristics of the most frequent conditions that can imitate oral infectious diseases in patients undergoing HCT.

Mucositis, once indistinct from HSV-related ulcers, is a conditioning regimen–related mucosal injury that presents 7 to 14 days after the initiation of conditioning and lasts for a median of 6 days, and is characterized by nonspecific irregular ulcerations that are restricted to the nonkeratinized mucosa.[31,144] Mucositis occurs in upward of 75% of patients undergoing myeloablative HCT, and importantly, lesions can become heavily colonized by the oral flora and may act as a portal of entry into the bloodstream.[145,146] Mucositis is not an infectious condition and antimicrobial prophylaxis regimens have no impact on its incidence.[145,147] It has been postulated that reducing mucositis may be an effective approach to reducing bloodstream infections.[16] Palifermin (Kepivance; keratinocyte growth factor) is the only agent approved by the Food and Drug Administration (FDA) for the prevention of mucositis in patients undergoing myeloablative HCT.[148,149]

Acute GVHD infrequently presents with oral findings characterized by nonspecific erythema and ulceration that are typically associated with more classic skin and gut findings and occur after engraftment, following resolution of mucositis.[150] Patients receiving sirolimus-containing GVHD prophylaxis regimens may be at risk for developing aphthous-like oral ulcers in the post-transplantation period.[151]

Diagnostic Studies

Empiric therapy based on clinical characteristics can be initiated in many cases, especially in the case of pseudomembranous candidiasis where clinical diagnosis is usually adequate and positive culture results do not confirm clinical infection.[152] Similarly, oral ulcerations that are consistent with mucositis are not typically cultured because acyclovir prophylaxis is highly effective. The routine diagnostic procedure for detecting HSV in oral lesions is viral culture, and positive samples can be tested for antiviral susceptibility when resistance is suspected. Viral cultures must be delivered to the laboratory within 1 hour to minimize false-negative results, and it typically takes 2 or more days to confirm diagnosis.[153] Cytopathology can provide a more rapid diagnosis of HSV and candidiasis, although the procedure is more invasive and more uncomfortable for the patient compared with swabbing for a culture.[153,154] To absolutely rule out HSV infection, especially in the context of a negative viral culture, tissue biopsy is necessary, and positive viral cytopathic changes can be confirmed with immunohistochemical staining for HSV-1. Deep fungal infections may be initially detected by serum glucan and galactomannan antigen testing; however, tissue biopsy of a suspected oral lesion is required to confirm the diagnosis.[93,155] Odontogenic infections can typically be diagnosed by standard clinical and radiographic evaluation.

Treatment During Neutropenia

Treatment of odontogenic infections during neutropenia and thrombocytopenia is usually carried out with antibacterials and analgesics while deferring potentially invasive definitive procedures (eg, extraction) until after recovery of blood counts. Patients with platelet counts less than 50,000 cells/μL should ideally be transfused before invasive interventions, although adequate hemostasis can usually be achieved after simple extractions and small biopsies at levels as low as 10 to 20,000/μL.[156]

ANTIVIRAL AGENTS
Nucleoside Analogues

Since its clinical introduction 30 years ago, acyclovir has been the first-line treatment for

HSV infections.[12] Acyclovir is selectively phosphorylated in virally infected cells by viral thymidine kinase (TK) and cellular kinases in the cytoplasm, after which its potent derivative acyclovir triphosphate is transported into the nucleus, where it inhibits viral DNA polymerase.[157–159] The low bioavailability of acyclovir led to the development of valacyclovir, which has approximately 10-fold (6% vs 60%) the bioavailability of acyclovir. Famciclovir (Famvir), the oral prodrug of penciclovir (Denavir), has even higher bioavailability than valacyclovir, but requires twice as high concentrations to obtain the same inhibitory effect in vitro. Although in vivo effects have been demonstrated, it is only approved against VZV.[12,160] Breakthrough lesions that occur during low-dose acyclovir prophylaxis can usually be managed with valacyclovir or famciclovir, or by simply increasing the dose intensity of acyclovir.

Resistance to acyclovir is exceedingly rare in the immunocompetent population; however, resistance in immunocompromised patients has been reported to range from 6% to 7%.[161–163] Most mutations are identified in viral TK (95% of all resistant strains), with the remainder occurring in viral DNA polymerase.[164,165] Nevertheless, a recent case series reports the effectiveness of continuous infusion of high-dose acyclovir against resistant strains.[166]

Other Antiviral Agents

Foscarnet (Foscavir) and cidofovir (Vistide) are intravenous antiviral agents that have efficacy against HSV infections that are resistant to nucleoside analogues.[167,168] Because neither is dependent on viral TK phosphorylation, both are usually effective against resistant strains that have undergone TK mutations.[12,169] In one study of 20 acyclovir-resistant HSV strains, all demonstrated cross-resistance to penciclovir, three showed resistance to foscarnet, and all were susceptible to cidofovir.[164] The two major shortcomings of foscarnet and cidofovir are low bioavailability and nephrotoxicity; therefore, both agents are only available in intravenous formulation and generally require inpatient management with careful monitoring of fluids and electrolytes.[170,171] Although cidofovir has a longer half-life and can be more convenient for outpatients, foscarnet is usually the first choice because it is less nephrotoxic.

ANTIFUNGAL AGENTS
Topical Treatment

Treatment of oral candidiasis can be achieved with topical or systemic antifungal agents, with the choice depending on several factors including severity of the disease, need for long-term administration, organ dysfunction, and drug interactions. Widely used topical regimens include nystatin suspension and clotrimazole troches, both of which bind to the fungal membrane and alter permeability.[172] Nystatin is a polyene antifungal agent that is toxic when given systemically, but is not absorbed through the gut when swallowed, thus permitting safe and effective topical management of oral, oropharyngeal, and esophageal candidiasis.[173–175] Nystatin is also formulated in an ointment or cream and is effective in the management of angular cheilitis, especially when combined with triamcinolone (Mycolog II). Clotrimazole is an azole antifungal with fungistatic activity and anti-staphylococcal activity and is also ideal against angular cheilitis as an ointment, as well as oral candidiasis.[176] Clotrimazole troches dissolve in the mouth and bind to the mucosa from where it is slowly released, and although systemic absorption is thought to be minimal, like the other azoles it is a cytochrome P-450 inhibitor and may result in elevated serum levels of several drugs (**Table 2**).[177,178]

Other topical agents include miconazole buccal tablets (Oravig), which have been shown to be as effective as clotrimazole and may be effective in cases of resistance to other azoles.[179] Amphotericin B (AmBisome), a polyene that is available as a topical rinse, has been found to be effective in azole-refractory oral candidiasis.[180] Chlorhexidine gluconate rinse is a commonly used antimicrobial agent that has considerable antifungal activity but cannot be swallowed.[181]

Systemic Treatment

The most widely used systemic antifungal agents are from the azole and polyene classes. In immunocompromised patients, systemic antifungal therapy has been shown to be more effective than topical therapy in reducing symptoms of candidiasis and eliminating *Candida* from the oral cavity.[182] In addition, severely immunocompromised patients may develop oral candidiasis despite topical antifungal prophylaxis, necessitating initiation of systemic therapy. In some cases systemic therapy may be necessary because of poor compliance with topical regimens caused by intolerance (taste or consistency); nausea; and inability to adhere to frequent dosing.

First-generation azoles (fluconazole and itraconazole) are commonly used as first-line agents for management of oropharyngeal candidiasis.[183] Fluconazole is generally highly effective against *C albicans*, although resistance does occur.[184]

Table 2
Interactions between azoles and frequently used drugs in HCT patients

Drugs with Significant Interactions	Azoles with Available Data	Effects
Cyclosporine	Ketaconazole > voriconazole, itraconazole > fluconazole	Increased concentration of cyclosporine
Tacrolimus	Ketaconazole > voriconazole, itraconazole > fluconazole	Increased concentration of tacrolimus
Sirolimus	Ketaconazole > voriconazole, itraconazole > fluconazole	Increased concentration of sirolimus
Corticosteroids	Itraconazole	Increased concentration of corticosteroids
Cyclophosphamide	Itraconazole	Increased concentration of cyclophosphamide
Busulfan	Itraconazole (not fluconazole)	Increased concentration of busulfan
Vincristine	Itraconazole	Increased concentration of vincristine
Vinca alkaloids	Voriconazole, posaconazole	Increased concentration of vinca alkaloid
Anthracyclines	Azoles	Prolonged QT interval[a]
Rifamycins (rifampin, rifabutin)	Itraconazole, posaconazole	Increased concentration of rifamycin

[a] Case reports linking prolonged QT interval with administering azoles shortly after anthracycline treatment have been published. Azoles are therefore not given until a minimum of 24 hours after the last anthracycline dose in many clinical trials.

Adapted from Dodds-Ashley E. Management of drug and food interactions with azole antifungal agents in transplant recipients. Pharmacotherapy 2010;30(8):842–54; with permission.

The greatest limitation of fluconazole is that other Candidal species (eg, *C krusei, C glabrata,* and *C dubliniensis*) are frequently resistant, and it has no activity against molds (eg. *Aspergillus, Zygomycetes,* and *Fusarium*).[185,186] Although itraconazole might be more effective and has a wider spectrum than fluconazole with some activity against *Aspergillus,* it is more commonly associated with hepatic and renal dysfunction.[187] Voriconazole (VFEND) and posaconazole are often effective in cases that are resistant to first-generation azoles, although cross-resistance can occur.[188] Because of increasing azole resistance in various fungal species in neutropenic patients, recent guidelines recommend that azoles should be avoided as an empiric therapy if already used for prophylaxis.[189,190]

As with clotrimazole, all systemic azoles are cytochrome P-450 inhibitors and must be used with caution in combination with several agents often used in HCT recipients, such as cyclosporine, corticosteroids, tacrolimus, and sirolimus (see **Table 2**).[191] Itraconazole and voriconazole are also cytochrome P-450 substrates, therefore their levels can be altered when coadministered with a number of drugs.[191] In addition to this, itraconazole, posaconazole, and ketoconazole are P-glycoprotein (P-gp) inhibitors. Often interactions involve both mechanisms, as is the case with several immunosuppressive (eg, cyclosporine, tacrolimus, and sirolimus) and antineoplastic agents (vincristine, vinblastine, doxorubicin, paclotaxel, and etoposide).[191,192] It should also be noted that fluconazole, itraconazole, and posaconazole are P-gp substrates and their levels can be increased when coadministered with P-gp inhibitors. Importantly, the levels of these azoles are also decreased when used with P-gp inducers (eg, rifampin).[191,192] These drugs should not be administered without discussing drug interactions with the referring oncologist, proactively adjusting drug dosing, and making a clear monitoring plan to avoid toxicity.

Amphotericin B is generally effective against azole-resistant oropharyngeal candidiasis and most mold infections, and resistance is rare.[193] Nephrotoxicity is a concern, although the risk of this complication is reduced with lipid amphotericin B formulations.[194] Echinocandins (caspofungin, micafungin, and anidulafungin) are approved by the FDA for esophageal and other select forms of candidiasis and are increasingly used in cases of refractory oropharyngeal candidiasis, although there may be decreased sensitivity to *C parapsilosis*, *C krusei*, and *C glabrata*.[195] Caspofungin is approved by the FDA for empiric therapy of febrile neutropenia.[138] The echinocandins are equally as effective as amphotericin B while being much less toxic. Unlike the azoles, echinocandins rarely interact with other drugs.[138,185,196]

Deep fungal infections in the oral cavity are rare but prompt diagnosis and aggressive therapy can significantly increase survival rates.[197] Management includes surgical debridement when applicable and intensive antifungal therapy with amphotericin B, voriconazole, or posaconazole, plus reduction of systemic immunosuppressive therapy when appropriate.[198]

ANTIBACTERIAL AGENTS

Given the increasing incidence of penicillin resistance the use of amoxicillin combined with clavulanic acid (Augmentin) has been recommended for odontogenic infections in severely immunocompromised patients.[199,200] However, one study in 103 patients who underwent surgical incision and drainage showed similar high susceptibility rates of viridans streptococci to penicillins and clindamycin (87% and 86% respectively) suggesting that these can be used as initial empiric therapy for odontogenic infections.[200] The most frequently resistant oral species are from the *Prevotella* group with the most frequent mechanism of resistance being the formation of β-lactamases usually inhibited by the addition of clavulanic acid.[107] When enhanced activity against anaerobes is required as in necrotizing gingivitis and other advanced periodontal infections the addition of metronidazole (Flagyl) should be considered.[201] In the case of suspected gram-positive bacteremia, vancomycin (Vancocin) is initiated empirically until susceptibility is known.[172]

SUMMARY

This article reviews the most frequent infectious oral complications in patients undergoing HCT and others who are severely immunocompromised. Prevention, accurate and timely diagnosis, and effective and often aggressive management approaches with careful follow-up are critical in minimizing morbidity and improving treatment outcomes. Optimal management of these patients benefits greatly from interdisciplinary consultation and communication between oral medicine and infectious disease specialists and the primary oncology medical team.

REFERENCES

1. Hansen JA, Clift RA, Thomas ED, et al. Transplantation of marrow from an unrelated donor to a patient with acute leukemia. N Engl J Med 1980;303(10):565–7.
2. Jenq RR, van den Brink MR. Allogeneic haematopoietic stem cell transplantation: individualized stem cell and immune therapy of cancer. Nat Rev Cancer 2010;10(3):213–21.
3. Lark RL, McNeil SA, VanderHyde K, et al. Risk factors for anaerobic bloodstream infections in bone marrow transplant recipients. Clin Infect Dis 2001;33(3):338–43.
4. Mikulska M, Del Bono V, Raiola AM, et al. Blood stream infections in allogeneic hematopoietic stem cell transplant recipients: reemergence of gram-negative rods and increasing antibiotic resistance. Biol Blood Marrow Transplant 2009;15(1):47–53.
5. Storek J. Immunological reconstitution after hematopoietic cell transplantation: its relation to the contents of the graft. Expert Opin Biol Ther 2008;8(5):583–97.
6. Joseph RW, Couriel DR, Komanduri KV. Chronic graft-versus-host disease after allogeneic stem cell transplantation: challenges in prevention, science, and supportive care. J Support Oncol 2008;6(8):361–72.
7. Devetten MP, Hari PN, Carreras J, et al. Unrelated donor reduced-intensity allogeneic hematopoietic stem cell transplantation for relapsed and refractory Hodgkin lymphoma. Biol Blood Marrow Transplant 2009;15(1):109–17.
8. Mikulska M, Del Bono V, Prinapori R, et al. Risk factors for enterococcal bacteremia in allogeneic hematopoietic stem cell transplant recipients. Transpl Infect Dis 2010;12(6):505–12.
9. Gooley TA, Chien JW, Pergam SA, et al. Reduced mortality after allogeneic hematopoietic-cell transplantation. N Engl J Med 2010;363(22):2091–101.
10. Morschhauser J. The genetic basis of fluconazole resistance development in *Candida albicans*. Biochim Biophys Acta 2002;1587(2–3):240–8.
11. Ortega M, Rovira M, Almela M, et al. Bacterial and fungal bloodstream isolates from 796 hematopoietic stem cell transplant recipients between 1991 and 2000. Ann Hematol 2005;84(1):40–6.
12. Piret J, Boivin G. Resistance of herpes simplex viruses to nucleoside analogues: mechanisms, prevalence and management. Antimicrob Agents Chemother 2011;55(2):459–72.

13. Eisen D, Essell J, Broun ER. Oral cavity complications of bone marrow transplantation. Semin Cutan Med Surg 1997;16(4):265–72.

14. Cunha BA, Eisenstein LE, Dillard T, et al. Herpes simplex virus (HSV) pneumonia in a heart transplant: diagnosis and therapy. Heart Lung 2007; 36(1):72–8.

15. Holley A, Dulhunty J, Blot S, et al. Temporal trends, risk factors and outcomes in albicans and non-albicans candidaemia: an international epidemiological study in four multidisciplinary intensive care units. Int J Antimicrob Agents 2009;33(6): 554, e551–7.

16. Scully C, Sonis S, Diz PD. Oral mucositis. Oral Dis 2006;12(3):229–41.

17. Brady RC, Bernstein DI. Treatment of herpes simplex virus infections. Antiviral Res 2004;61(2): 73–81.

18. Halioua B, Malkin JE. Epidemiology of genital herpes: recent advances. Eur J Dermatol 1999; 9(3):177–84.

19. Lafferty WE, Coombs RW, Benedetti J, et al. Recurrences after oral and genital herpes simplex virus infection. N Engl J Med 1987;316(23):1444–9.

20. Langenberg AG, Corey L, Ashley RL, et al. A prospective study of new infections with herpes simplex virus type 1 and type 2. Chiron HSV Vaccine Study Group. N Engl J Med 1999; 341(19):1432–8.

21. Xu F, Sternberg MR, Kottiri BJ, et al. Trends in herpes simplex virus type 1 and type 2 seroprevalence in the United States. JAMA 2006; 296(8):964–73.

22. Holbrook WP, Gudmundsson GT, Ragnarsson KT. Herpetic gingivostomatitis in otherwise healthy adolescents and young adults. Acta Odontol Scand 2001;59(3):113–5.

23. Katz J, Marmary I, Ben-Yehuda A, et al. Primary herpetic gingivostomatitis: no longer a disease of childhood? Community Dent Oral Epidemiol 1991; 19(5):309.

24. Miller CS, Danaher RJ, Jacob RJ. Molecular aspects of herpes simplex virus I latency, reactivation, and recurrence. Crit Rev Oral Biol Med 1998; 9(4):541–62.

25. Young SK, Rowe NH, Buchanan RA. A clinical study for the control of facial mucocutaneous herpes virus infections. I. Characterization of natural history in a professional school population. Oral Surg Oral Med Oral Pathol 1976;41(4):498–507.

26. Embil JA, Stephens RG, Manuel FR. Prevalence of recurrent herpes labialis and aphthous ulcers among young adults on six continents. Can Med Assoc J 1975;113(7):627–30.

27. Knaup B, Schunemann S, Wolff MH. Subclinical reactivation of herpes simplex virus type 1 in the oral cavity. Oral Microbiol Immunol 2000;15(5):281–3.

28. Stanberry LR, Cunningham AL, Mindel A, et al. Prospects for control of herpes simplex virus disease through immunization. Clin Infect Dis 2000;30(3):549–66.

29. Cohen SG, Greenberg MS. Chronic oral herpes simplex virus infection in immunocompromised patients. Oral Surg Oral Med Oral Pathol 1985; 59(5):465–71.

30. Woo SB, Lee SF. Oral recrudescent herpes simplex virus infection. Oral Surg Oral Med Oral Pathol Oral Radiol Endod 1997;83(2):239–43.

31. Bergmann OJ, Mogensen SC, Ellegaard J. Herpes simplex virus and intraoral ulcers in immunocompromised patients with haematologic malignancies. Eur J Clin Microbiol Infect Dis 1990;9(3):184–90.

32. Smyth RL, Higenbottam TW, Scott JP, et al. Herpes simplex virus infection in heart-lung transplant recipients. Transplantation 1990;49(4):735–9.

33. Ramsey PG, Fife KH, Hackman RC, et al. Herpes simplex virus pneumonia: clinical, virologic, and pathologic features in 20 patients. Ann Intern Med 1982;97(6):813–20.

34. Romee R, Brunstein CG, Weisdorf DJ, et al. Herpes simplex virus encephalitis after allogeneic transplantation: an instructive case. Bone Marrow Transplant 2010;45(4):776–8.

35. Whitley RJ. Herpes simplex virus infections of the central nervous system. Encephalitis and neonatal herpes. Drugs 1991;42(3):406–27.

36. Locksley RM, Flournoy N, Sullivan KM, et al. Infection with varicella-zoster virus after marrow transplantation. J Infect Dis 1985;152(6):1172–81.

37. Boeckh M, Kim HW, Flowers ME, et al. Long-term acyclovir for prevention of varicella zoster virus disease after allogeneic hematopoietic cell transplantation–a randomized double-blind placebo-controlled study. Blood 2006;107(5):1800–5.

38. Ragozzino MW, Melton LJ, Kurland LT, et al. Population-based study of herpes zoster and its sequelae. Medicine (Baltimore) 1982;61(5):310–6.

39. Schmidt-Hieber M, Schwender J, Heinz W, et al. Viral encephalitis after allogeneic stem cell transplantation: a rare complication with distinct characteristics of different causative agents. Haematologica 2011; 96(1):142–9.

40. Feldman S, Lott L. Varicella in children with cancer: impact of antiviral therapy and prophylaxis. Pediatrics 1987;80(4):465–72.

41. Mendieta C, Miranda J, Brunet LI, et al. Alveolar bone necrosis and tooth exfoliation following herpes zoster infection: a review of the literature and case report. J Periodontol 2005;76(1):148–53.

42. Munoz-Sellart M, Garcia-Vidal C, Martinez-Yelamos S, et al. Peripheral facial palsy after varicella. Report of two cases and review of the literature. Enferm Infecc Microbiol Clin 2010; 28(8):504–8.

43. Ter Meulen BC, Rath JJ. Motor radiculopathy caused by varicella zoster virus without skin lesions ('zoster sine herpete'). Clin Neurol Neurosurg 2010; 112(10):933.

44. Lackner A, Kessler HH, Walch C, et al. Early and reliable detection of herpes simplex virus type 1 and varicella zoster virus DNAs in oral fluid of patients with idiopathic peripheral facial nerve palsy: decision support regarding antiviral treatment? J Med Virol 2010;82(9):1582–5.

45. Onozawa M, Hashino S, Haseyama Y, et al. Incidence and risk of postherpetic neuralgia after varicella zoster virus infection in hematopoietic cell transplantation recipients: Hokkaido Hematology Study Group. Biol Blood Marrow Transplant 2009; 15(6):724–9.

46. Goh CL, Khoo L. A retrospective study on the clinical outcome of herpes zoster in patients treated with acyclovir or valaciclovir vs. patients not treated with antiviral. Int J Dermatol 1998;37(7):544–6.

47. Oxman MN, Levin MJ, Johnson GR, et al. A vaccine to prevent herpes zoster and postherpetic neuralgia in older adults. N Engl J Med 2005;352(22):2271–84.

48. Opelz G, Henderson R. Incidence of non-Hodgkin lymphoma in kidney and heart transplant recipients. Lancet 1993;342(8886–8887):1514–6.

49. Curtis RE, Travis LB, Rowlings PA, et al. Risk of lymphoproliferative disorders after bone marrow transplantation: a multi-institutional study. Blood 1999; 94(7):2208–16.

50. Pickhardt PJ, Siegel MJ, Hayashi RJ, et al. Posttransplantation lymphoproliferative disorder in children: clinical, histopathologic, and imaging features. Radiology 2000;217(1):16–25.

51. Elad S, Meyerowitz C, Shapira MY, et al. Oral posttransplantation lymphoproliferative disorder: an uncommon site for an uncommon disorder. Oral Surg Oral Med Oral Pathol Oral Radiol Endod 2008;105(1):59–64.

52. Ballen KK, Cutler C, Yeap BY, et al. Donor-derived second hematologic malignancies after cord blood transplantation. Biol Blood Marrow Transplant 2010;16(7):1025–31.

53. Styczynski J, Einsele H, Gil L, et al. Outcome of treatment of Epstein-Barr virus-related posttransplant lymphoproliferative disorder in hematopoietic stem cell recipients: a comprehensive review of reported cases. Transpl Infect Dis 2009; 11(5):383–92.

54. Thomas JA, Crawford DH, Burke M. Clinicopathologic implications of Epstein-Barr virus related B cell lymphoma in immunocompromised patients. J Clin Pathol 1995;48(4):287–90.

55. Manez R, Breinig MC, Linden P, et al. Posttransplant lymphoproliferative disease in primary Epstein-Barr virus infection after liver transplantation: the role of cytomegalovirus disease. J Infect Dis 1997;176(6): 1462–7.

56. Haque T, Thomas JA, Falk KI, et al. Transmission of donor Epstein-Barr virus (EBV) in transplanted organs causes lymphoproliferative disease in EBV-seronegative recipients. J Gen Virol 1996; 77(Pt 6):1169–72.

57. Ho M, Jaffe R, Miller G, et al. The frequency of Epstein-Barr virus infection and associated lymphoproliferative syndrome after transplantation and its manifestations in children. Transplantation 1988;45(4):719–27.

58. Ho M, Miller G, Atchison RW, et al. Epstein-Barr virus infections and DNA hybridization studies in posttransplantation lymphoma and lymphoproliferative lesions: the role of primary infection. J Infect Dis 1985;152(5):876–86.

59. DiNardo CD, Tsai DE. Treatment advances in posttransplant lymphoproliferative disease. Curr Opin Hematol 2010;17(4):368–74.

60. Johnson J, Kerecuk L, Harrison M, et al. Epstein-Barr virus-associated lymphoproliferative disease in oral cavity in a renal transplant recipient: a case report. Pediatr Transplant 2007;11(3):340–4.

61. Wilde GE, Moore DJ, Bellah RD. Posttransplantation lymphoproliferative disorder in pediatric recipients of solid organ transplants: timing and location of disease. AJR Am J Roentgenol 2005;185(5): 1335–41.

62. Kerkar N, Morotti RA, Madan RP, et al. The changing face of post-transplant lymphoproliferative disease in the era of molecular EBV monitoring. Pediatr Transplant 2010;14(4):504–11.

63. Martin JM, Danziger-Isakov LA. Cytomegalovirus risk, prevention, and management in pediatric solid organ transplantation. Pediatr Transplant 2011; 15(3):229–36.

64. Bate SL, Dollard SC, Cannon MJ. Cytomegalovirus seroprevalence in the United States: the national health and nutrition examination surveys, 1988-2004. Clin Infect Dis 2010;50(11):1439–47.

65. Correia-Silva Jde F, Victoria JM, Guimaraes AL, et al. Cytomegalovirus shedding in the oral cavity of allogeneic haematopoietic stem cell transplant patients. Oral Dis 2007;13(2):163–9.

66. Ammatuna P, Campisi G, Giovannelli L, et al. Presence of Epstein-Barr virus, cytomegalovirus and human papillomavirus in normal oral mucosa of HIV-infected and renal transplant patients. Oral Dis 2001;7(1):34–40.

67. Saral R, Burns WH, Prentice HG. Herpes virus infections: clinical manifestations and therapeutic strategies in immunocompromised patients. Clin Haematol 1984;13(3):645–60.

68. Boeckh M, Leisenring W, Riddell SR, et al. Late cytomegalovirus disease and mortality in recipients of allogeneic hematopoietic stem cell

transplants: importance of viral load and T-cell immunity. Blood 2003;101(2):407–14.

69. Farahani RM, Marsee DK, Baden LR, et al. Trigeminal trophic syndrome with features of oral CMV disease. Oral Surg Oral Med Oral Pathol Oral Radiol Endod 2008;106(3):e15–8.

70. Luppi M, Barozzi P, Rasini V, et al. HHV-8 infection in the transplantation setting: a concern only for solid organ transplant patients? Leuk Lymphoma 2002;43(3):517–22.

71. Qu L, Jenkins F, Triulzi DJ. Human herpesvirus 8 genomes and seroprevalence in United States blood donors. Transfusion 2010;50(5):1050–6.

72. Lazzi S, Bellan C, Amato T, et al. Kaposi's sarcoma-associated herpesvirus/human herpesvirus 8 infection in reactive lymphoid tissues: a model for KSHV/HHV-8-related lymphomas? Hum Pathol 2006;37(1):23–31.

73. Marcen R, Galeano C, Fernandez-Rodriguez A, et al. Effects of the new immunosuppressive agents on the occurrence of malignancies after renal transplantation. Transplant Proc 2010;42(8):3055–7.

74. Stefan DC, Stones DK, Wainwright L, et al. Kaposi sarcoma in South African children. Pediatr Blood Cancer 2011;56(3):392–6.

75. Marco de F, Infante B, Giovanni S, et al. Rapamycin for Kaposi's sarcoma and graft-versus-host disease in bone marrow transplant recipient. Transplantation 2010;89(5):633–4.

76. Shiboski CH, Patton LL, Webster-Cyriaque JY, et al. The Oral HIV/AIDS Research Alliance: updated case definitions of oral disease endpoints. J Oral Pathol Med 2009;38(6):481–8.

77. Castro TP, Bussoloti Filho I. Prevalence of human papillomavirus (HPV) in oral cavity and oropharynx. Braz J Otorhinolaryngol 2006;72(2):272–82.

78. Zeuss MS, Miller CS, White DK. In situ hybridization analysis of human papillomavirus DNA in oral mucosal lesions. Oral Surg Oral Med Oral Pathol 1991;71(6):714–20.

79. Zhao D, Xu QG, Chen XM, et al. Human papillomavirus as an independent predictor in oral squamous cell cancer. Int J Oral Sci 2009;1(3):119–25.

80. Lewis DM. Verrucous oral lesions: possibly not so innocuous after all. Squamous papilloma. J Okla Dent Assoc 2009;100(5):18–20.

81. Cho HK, Lee NY, Lee H, et al. Enterovirus 71-associated hand, foot and mouth diseases with neurologic symptoms, a university hospital experience in Korea, 2009. Korean J Pediatr 2010;53(5):639–43.

82. Scully C, el-Kabir M, Samaranayake LP. Candida and oral candidosis: a review. Crit Rev Oral Biol Med 1994;5(2):125–57.

83. Zomorodian K, Haghighi NN, Rajaee N, et al. Assessment of Candida species colonization and denture-related stomatitis in complete denture wearers. Med Mycol 2011;49(2):208–11.

84. Schorling SR, Kortinga HC, Froschb M, et al. The role of Candida dubliniensis in oral candidiasis in human immunodeficiency virus-infected individuals. Crit Rev Microbiol 2000;26(1):59–68.

85. Sullivan DJ, Westerneng TJ, Haynes KA, et al. Candida dubliniensis sp. nov.: phenotypic and molecular characterization of a novel species associated with oral candidosis in HIV-infected individuals. Microbiology 1995;141(Pt 7):1507–21.

86. Meis JF, Ruhnke M, De Pauw BE, et al. Candida dubliniensis candidemia in patients with chemotherapy-induced neutropenia and bone marrow transplantation. Emerg Infect Dis 1999;5(1): 150–3.

87. Odds FC, Kibbler CC, Walker E, et al. Carriage of Candida species and C albicans biotypes in patients undergoing chemotherapy or bone marrow transplantation for haematological disease. J Clin Pathol 1989;42(12):1259–66.

88. Kiehn TE, Edwards FF, Armstrong D. The prevalence of yeasts in clinical specimens from cancer patients. Am J Clin Pathol 1980;73(4):518–21.

89. Pereira HA, Hosking CS. The role of complement and antibody in opsonization and intracellular killing of Candida albicans. Clin Exp Immunol 1984;57(2):307–14.

90. Papadimitriou JM, Ashman RB. Macrophages: current views on their differentiation, structure, and function. Ultrastruct Pathol 1989;13(4):343–72.

91. Epstein JB, Kimura LH, Menard TW, et al. Effects of specific antibodies on the interaction between the fungus Candida albicans and human oral mucosa. Arch Oral Biol 1982;27(6):469–74.

92. Samaranayake LP, Keung Leung W, Jin L. Oral mucosal fungal infections. Periodontol 2000 2009; 49:39–59.

93. Michallet M, Ito JI. Approaches to the management of invasive fungal infections in hematologic malignancy and hematopoietic cell transplantation. J Clin Oncol 2009;27(20):3398–409.

94. Marr KA, Seidel K, White TC, et al. Candidemia in allogeneic blood and marrow transplant recipients: evolution of risk factors after the adoption of prophylactic fluconazole. J Infect Dis 2000; 181(1):309–16.

95. DeGregorio MW, Lee WM, Ries CA. Candida infections in patients with acute leukemia: ineffectiveness of nystatin prophylaxis and relationship between oropharyngeal and systemic candidiasis. Cancer 1982;50(12):2780–4.

96. Gautam H, Kaur R, Goyal R, et al. Oral thrush to candidemia: a morbid outcome. J Int Assoc Physicians AIDS Care (Chic) 2010;9(5):325–7.

97. Fuqua TH Jr, Sittitavornwong S, Knoll M, et al. Primary invasive oral aspergillosis: an updated literature review. J Oral Maxillofac Surg 2010; 68(10):2557–63.

98. Cho H, Lee KH, Colquhoun AN, et al. Invasive oral aspergillosis in a patient with acute myeloid leukaemia. Aust Dent J 2010;55(2):214–8.

99. Myoken Y, Sugata T, Kyo TI, et al. Pathological features of invasive oral aspergillosis in patients with hematologic malignancies. J Oral Maxillofac Surg 1996;54(3):263–70.

100. Jantunen E, Nihtinen A, Anttila VJ. Changing landscape of invasive aspergillosis in allogeneic stem cell transplant recipients. Transpl Infect Dis 2008; 10(3):156–61.

101. Neofytos D, Horn D, Anaissie E, et al. Epidemiology and outcome of invasive fungal infection in adult hematopoietic stem cell transplant recipients: analysis of Multicenter Prospective Antifungal Therapy (PATH) Alliance registry. Clin Infect Dis 2009; 48(3):265–73.

102. Perkhofer S, Lass-Florl C, Hell M, et al. The Nationwide Austrian Aspergillus Registry: a prospective data collection on epidemiology, therapy and outcome of invasive mould infections in immunocompromised and/or immunosuppressed patients. Int J Antimicrob Agents 2010;36(6):531–6.

103. McDermott NE, Barrett J, Hipp J, et al. Successful treatment of periodontal mucormycosis: report of a case and literature review. Oral Surg Oral Med Oral Pathol Oral Radiol Endod 2010;109(3):e64–9.

104. Graber CJ, de Almeida KN, Atkinson JC, et al. Dental health and *Viridans* streptococcal bacteremia in allogeneic hematopoietic stem cell transplant recipients. Bone Marrow Transplant 2001; 27(5):537–42.

105. Kuderer NM, Dale DC, Crawford J, et al. Mortality, morbidity, and cost associated with febrile neutropenia in adult cancer patients. Cancer 2006; 106(10):2258–66.

106. Sparrelid E, Hagglund H, Remberger M, et al. Bacteraemia during the aplastic phase after allogeneic bone marrow transplantation is associated with early death from invasive fungal infection. Bone Marrow Transplant 1998;22(8):795–800.

107. Robertson D, Smith AJ. The microbiology of the acute dental abscess. J Med Microbiol 2009; 58(Pt 2):155–62.

108. Bresco-Salinas M, Costa-Riu N, Berini-Aytes L, et al. Antibiotic susceptibility of the bacteria causing odontogenic infections. Med Oral Patol Oral Cir Bucal 2006;11(1):E70–5.

109. Huang TT, Tseng FY, Yeh TH, et al. Factors affecting the bacteriology of deep neck infection: a retrospective study of 128 patients. Acta Otolaryngol 2006;126(4):396–401.

110. Hancock HH 3rd, Sigurdsson A, Trope M, et al. Bacteria isolated after unsuccessful endodontic treatment in a North American population. Oral Surg Oral Med Oral Pathol Oral Radiol Endod 2001;91(5):579–86.

111. Chow AW, Roser SM, Brady FA. Orofacial odontogenic infections. Ann Intern Med 1978;88(3):392–402.

112. Slutzky-Goldberg I, Tsesis I, Slutzky H, et al. Odontogenic sinus tracts: a cohort study. Quintessence Int 2009;40(1):13–8.

113. Reynolds SC, Chow AW. Life-threatening infections of the peripharyngeal and deep fascial spaces of the head and neck. Infect Dis Clin North Am 2007;21(2):557–76.

114. Raber-Durlacher JE, Epstein JB, Raber J, et al. Periodontal infection in cancer patients treated with high-dose chemotherapy. Support Care Cancer 2002;10(6):466–73.

115. Jimenez LM, Duque FL, Baer PN, et al. Necrotizing ulcerative periodontal diseases in children and young adults in Medellin, Colombia, 1965–2000. J Int Acad Periodontol 2005;7(2):55–63.

116. Falkler WA Jr, Enwonwu CO, Idigbe EO. Microbiological understandings and mysteries of noma (cancrum oris). Oral Dis 1999;5(2):150–5.

117. Horning GM, Cohen ME. Necrotizing ulcerative gingivitis, periodontitis, and stomatitis: clinical staging and predisposing factors. J Periodontol 1995;66(11):990–8.

118. von Wowern N, Nielsen HO. The fate of impacted lower third molars after the age of 20. A four-year clinical follow-up. Int J Oral Maxillofac Surg 1989; 18(5):277–80.

119. Ohman D, Bjork Y, Bratel J, et al. Partially erupted third molars as a potential source of infection in patients receiving peripheral stem cell transplantation for malignant diseases: a retrospective study. Eur J Oral Sci 2010;118(1):53–8.

120. Woo SB, Matin K. Off-site dental evaluation program for prospective bone marrow transplant recipients. J Am Dent Assoc 1997;128(2):189–93.

121. Yamagata K, Onizawa K, Yanagawa T, et al. Prospective study establishing a management plan for impacted third molar in patients undergoing hematopoietic stem cell transplantation. Oral Surg Oral Med Oral Pathol Oral Radiol Endod 2011;111(2):146–52.

122. Bishay N, Petrikowski CG, Maxymiw WG, et al. Optimum dental radiography in bone marrow transplant patients. Oral Surg Oral Med Oral Pathol Oral Radiol Endod 1999;87(3):375–9.

123. Peters E, Monopoli M, Woo SB, et al. Assessment of the need for treatment of postendodontic asymptomatic periapical radiolucencies in bone marrow transplant recipients. Oral Surg Oral Med Oral Pathol 1993;76(1):45–8.

124. Weikel DS, Peterson DE, Rubinstein LE, et al. Incidence of fever following invasive oral interventions in the myelosuppressed cancer patient. Cancer Nurs 1989;12(5):265–70.

125. Antunes HS, Ferreira EM, de Faria LM, et al. Streptococcal bacteraemia in patients submitted to

hematopoietic stem cell transplantation: the role of tooth brushing and use of chlorhexidine. Med Oral Patol Oral Cir Bucal 2010;15(2):e303–9.

126. Center for International Blood and Marrow Transplant Research (CIBMTR), National Marrow Donor Program (NMDP), European Blood and Marrow Transplant Group (EBMT), et al. Guidelines for preventing infectious complications among hematopoietic cell transplant recipients: a global perspective. Bone Marrow Transplant 2009;44(8): 453–8.

127. Anderson H, Scarffe JH, Sutton RN, et al. Oral acyclovir prophylaxis against herpes simplex virus in non-Hodgkin lymphoma and acute lymphoblastic leukaemia patients receiving remission induction chemotherapy. A randomised double blind, placebo controlled trial. Br J Cancer 1984; 50(1):45–9.

128. Saral R, Burns WH, Laskin OL, et al. Acyclovir prophylaxis of herpes-simplex-virus infections. N Engl J Med 1981;305(2):63–7.

129. Saral R, Ambinder RF, Burns WH, et al. Acyclovir prophylaxis against herpes simplex virus infection in patients with leukemia. A randomized, double-blind, placebo-controlled study. Ann Intern Med 1983;99(6):773–6.

130. Schubert MM, Peterson DE, Flournoy N, et al. Oral and pharyngeal herpes simplex virus infection after allogeneic bone marrow transplantation: analysis of factors associated with infection. Oral Surg Oral Med Oral Pathol 1990;70(3):286–93.

131. Dignani MC, Mykietiuk A, Michelet M, et al. Valacyclovir prophylaxis for the prevention of Herpes simplex virus reactivation in recipients of progenitor cells transplantation. Bone Marrow Transplant 2002;29(3):263–7.

132. Eisen D, Essell J, Broun ER, et al. Clinical utility of oral valacyclovir compared with oral acyclovir for the prevention of herpes simplex virus mucositis following autologous bone marrow transplantation or stem cell rescue therapy. Bone Marrow Transplant 2003;31(1):51–5.

133. Goodman JL, Winston DJ, Greenfield RA, et al. A controlled trial of fluconazole to prevent fungal infections in patients undergoing bone marrow transplantation. N Engl J Med 1992;326(13):845–51.

134. Winston DJ, Chandrasekar PH, Lazarus HM, et al. Fluconazole prophylaxis of fungal infections in patients with acute leukemia. Results of a randomized placebo-controlled, double-blind, multicenter trial. Ann Intern Med 1993;118(7):495–503.

135. Marr KA, Seidel K, Slavin MA, et al. Prolonged fluconazole prophylaxis is associated with persistent protection against candidiasis-related death in allogeneic marrow transplant recipients: long-term follow-up of a randomized, placebo-controlled trial. Blood 2000;96(6):2055–61.

136. Pfaller MA, Diekema DJ, Gibbs DL, et al. Results from the ARTEMIS DISK Global Antifungal Surveillance Study, 1997 to 2007: a 10.5-year analysis of susceptibilities of Candida Species to fluconazole and voriconazole as determined by CLSI standardized disk diffusion. J Clin Microbiol 2010;48(4): 1366–77.

137. Lyseng-Williamson KA. Posaconazole: a pharmacoeconomic review of its use in the prophylaxis of invasive fungal disease in immunocompromised hosts. Pharmacoeconomics 2011;29(3):251–68.

138. Chen SC, Slavin MA, Sorrell TC. Echinocandin antifungal drugs in fungal infections: a comparison. Drugs 2011;71(1):11–41.

139. Gafter-Gvili A, Fraser A, Paul M, et al. Meta-analysis: antibiotic prophylaxis reduces mortality in neutropenic patients. Ann Intern Med 2005; 142(12 Pt 1):979–95.

140. Bucaneve G, Micozzi A, Menichetti F, et al. Levofloxacin to prevent bacterial infection in patients with cancer and neutropenia. N Engl J Med 2005; 353(10):977–87.

141. MacDougall C, Powell JP, Johnson CK, et al. Hospital and community fluoroquinolone use and resistance in *Staphylococcus aureus* and *Escherichia coli* in 17 US hospitals. Clin Infect Dis 2005;41(4): 435–40.

142. Prabhu RM, Piper KE, Litzow MR, et al. Emergence of quinolone resistance among viridans group streptococci isolated from the oropharynx of neutropenic peripheral blood stem cell transplant patients receiving quinolone antimicrobial prophylaxis. Eur J Clin Microbiol Infect Dis 2005;24(12): 832–8.

143. Alcaide F, Linares J, Pallares R, et al. In vitro activities of 22 beta-lactam antibiotics against penicillin-resistant and penicillin-susceptible viridans group streptococci isolated from blood. Antimicrob Agents Chemother 1995;39(10):2243–7.

144. Redding SW. Role of herpes simplex virus reactivation in chemotherapy-induced oral mucositis. NCI Monogr 1990;(9):103–5.

145. Woo SB, Sonis ST, Monopoli MM, et al. A longitudinal study of oral ulcerative mucositis in bone marrow transplant recipients. Cancer 1993;72(5): 1612–7.

146. Sonis ST. Mucositis: the impact, biology and therapeutic opportunities of oral mucositis. Oral Oncol 2009;45(12):1015–20.

147. El-Sayed S, Nabid A, Shelley W, et al. Prophylaxis of radiation-associated mucositis in conventionally treated patients with head and neck cancer: a double-blind, phase III, randomized, controlled trial evaluating the clinical efficacy of an antimicrobial lozenge using a validated mucositis scoring system. J Clin Oncol 2002;20(19): 3956–63.

148. Sonis ST. Efficacy of palifermin (keratinocyte growth factor-1) in the amelioration of oral mucositis. Core Evid 2010;4:199–205.

149. Spielberger R, Stiff P, Bensinger W, et al. Palifermin for oral mucositis after intensive therapy for hematologic cancers. N Engl J Med 2004;351(25):2590–8.

150. Woo SB, Lee SJ, Schubert MM. Graft-vs.-host disease. Crit Rev Oral Biol Med 1997;8(2):201–16.

151. Sonis S, Treister N, Chawla S, et al. Preliminary characterization of oral lesions associated with inhibitors of mammalian target of rapamycin in cancer patients. Cancer 2010;116(1):210–5.

152. Mitchell KG, Bradley JA, Ledingham IM, et al. Candida colonization of the oral cavity. Surg Gynecol Obstet 1982;154(6):870–4.

153. Barrett AP, Buckley DJ, Greenberg ML, et al. The value of exfoliative cytology in the diagnosis of oral herpes simplex infection in immunosuppressed patients. Oral Surg Oral Med Oral Pathol 1986;62(2):175–8.

154. MacPhail LA, Hilton JF, Heinic GS, et al. Direct immunofluorescence vs. culture for detecting HSV in oral ulcers: a comparison. J Am Dent Assoc 1995;126(1):74–8.

155. Ruping MJ, Vehreschild JJ, Cornely OA. Patients at high risk of invasive fungal infections: when and how to treat. Drugs 2008;68(14):1941–62.

156. Williford SK, Salisbury PL, Peacock JE Jr, et al. The safety of dental extractions in patients with hematologic malignancies. J Clin Oncol 1989;7(6):798–802.

157. Miller WH, Miller RL. Phosphorylation of acyclovir (acycloguanosine) monophosphate by GMP kinase. J Biol Chem 1980;255(15):7204–7.

158. Reardon JE, Spector T. Herpes simplex virus type 1 DNA polymerase. Mechanism of inhibition by acyclovir triphosphate. J Biol Chem 1989;264(13):7405–11.

159. Miller WH, Miller RL. Phosphorylation of acyclovir diphosphate by cellular enzymes. Biochem Pharmacol 1982;31(23):3879–84.

160. Spruance SL, Rowe NH, Raborn GW, et al. Peroral famciclovir in the treatment of experimental ultraviolet radiation-induced herpes simplex labialis: a double-blind, dose-ranging, placebo-controlled, multicenter trial. J Infect Dis 1999;179(2):303–10.

161. Bacon TH, Boon RJ, Schultz M, et al. Surveillance for antiviral-agent-resistant herpes simplex virus in the general population with recurrent herpes labialis. Antimicrob Agents Chemother 2002;46(9):3042–4.

162. Christophers J, Clayton J, Craske J, et al. Survey of resistance of herpes simplex virus to acyclovir in northwest England. Antimicrob Agents Chemother 1998;42(4):868–72.

163. Chen Y, Scieux C, Garrait V, et al. Resistant herpes simplex virus type 1 infection: an emerging concern after allogeneic stem cell transplantation. Clin Infect Dis 2000;31(4):927–35.

164. Sauerbrei A, Deinhardt S, Zell R, et al. Phenotypic and genotypic characterization of acyclovir-resistant clinical isolates of herpes simplex virus. Antiviral Res 2010;86(3):246–52.

165. Elion GB, Furman PA, Fyfe JA, et al. The selectivity of action of an antiherpetic agent, 9-(2-hydroxyethoxymethyl) guanine. Reproduced from Proc. Natl. Acad. Sci. USA 74, 5716-5720 (1977). Rev Med Virol 1999;9(3):147–52 [discussion: 152–3].

166. Kim JH, Schaenman JM, Ho DY, et al. Treatment of acyclovir-resistant herpes simplex virus with continuous infusion of high-dose acyclovir in hematopoietic cell transplant patients. Biol Blood Marrow Transplant 2011;17(2):259–64.

167. Reusser P, Cordonnier C, Einsele H, et al. European survey of herpesvirus resistance to antiviral drugs in bone marrow transplant recipients. Infectious Diseases Working Party of the European Group for Blood and Marrow Transplantation (EBMT). Bone Marrow Transplant 1996;17(5):813–7.

168. Bronson JJ, Ghazzouli I, Hitchcock MJ, et al. Synthesis and antiviral activity of the nucleotide analogue (S)-1-[3-hydroxy-2-(phosphonylmethoxy)propyl]cytosine. J Med Chem 1989;32(7):1457–63.

169. Erlich KS, Jacobson MA, Koehler JE, et al. Foscarnet therapy for severe acyclovir-resistant herpes simplex virus type-2 infections in patients with the acquired immunodeficiency syndrome (AIDS). An uncontrolled trial. Ann Intern Med 1989;110(9):710–3.

170. Ringden O, Lonnqvist B, Paulin T, et al. Pharmacokinetics, safety and preliminary clinical experiences using foscarnet in the treatment of cytomegalovirus infections in bone marrow and renal transplant recipients. J Antimicrob Chemother 1986;17(3):373–87.

171. Wachsman M, Petty BG, Cundy KC, et al. Pharmacokinetics, safety and bioavailability of HPMPC (cidofovir) in human immunodeficiency virus-infected subjects. Antiviral Res 1996;29(2–3):153–61.

172. Lerman MA, Laudenbach J, Marty FM, et al. Management of oral infections in cancer patients. Dent Clin North Am 2008;52(1):129–53.

173. Austin N, Darlow BA, McGuire W. Prophylactic oral/topical non-absorbed antifungal agents to prevent invasive fungal infection in very low birth weight infants. Cochrane Database Syst Rev 2009;4:CD003478.

174. Badiee P, Alborzi A, Davarpanah MA, et al. Distributions and antifungal susceptibility of Candida species from mucosal sites in HIV positive patients. Arch Iran Med 2010;13(4):282–7.

175. Taylor TL. Nystatin prophylaxis in immunocompromised children. Ann Pharmacother 1996;30(5):534–5.

176. Alsterholm M, Karami N, Faergemann J. Antimicrobial activity of topical skin pharmaceuticals - an in vitro study. Acta Derm Venereol 2010;90(3):239–45.

177. Choy M. Tacrolimus interaction with clotrimazole: a concise case report and literature review. P T 2010;35(10):568–9.

178. Vasquez E, Pollak R, Benedetti E. Clotrimazole increases tacrolimus blood levels: a drug interaction in kidney transplant patients. Clin Transplant 2001;15(2):95–9.

179. Vazquez JA, Patton LL, Epstein JB, et al. Randomized, comparative, double-blind, double-dummy, multicenter trial of miconazole buccal tablet and clotrimazole troches for the treatment of oropharyngeal candidiasis: study of miconazole Lauriad(R) efficacy and safety (SMiLES). HIV Clin Trials 2010;11(4):186–96.

180. Grim SA, Smith KM, Romanelli F, et al. Treatment of azole-resistant oropharyngeal candidiasis with topical amphotericin B. Ann Pharmacother 2002; 36(9):1383–6.

181. Sritrairat N, Nukul N, Inthasame P, et al. Antifungal activity of lawsone methyl ether in comparison with chlorhexidine. J Oral Pathol Med 2011;40(1):90–6.

182. Pons V, Greenspan D, Debruin M. Therapy for oropharyngeal candidiasis in HIV-infected patients: a randomized, prospective multicenter study of oral fluconazole versus clotrimazole troches. The Multicenter Study Group. J Acquir Immune Defic Syndr 1993;6(12):1311–6.

183. Epstein JB, Truelove EL, Hanson-Huggins K, et al. Topical polyene antifungals in hematopoietic cell transplant patients: tolerability and efficacy. Support Care Cancer 2004;12(7):517–25.

184. Huang S, Cao YY, Dai BD, et al. In vitro synergism of fluconazole and baicalein against clinical isolates of *Candida albicans* resistant to fluconazole. Biol Pharm Bull 2008;31(12):2234–6.

185. Leather HL, Wingard JR. New strategies of antifungal therapy in hematopoietic stem cell transplant recipients and patients with hematological malignancies. Blood Rev 2006;20(5):267–87.

186. Wingard JR, Merz WG, Rinaldi MG, et al. Increase in *Candida krusei* infection among patients with bone marrow transplantation and neutropenia treated prophylactically with fluconazole. N Engl J Med 1991;325(18):1274–7.

187. Vardakas KZ, Michalopoulos A, Falagas ME. Fluconazole versus itraconazole for antifungal prophylaxis in neutropenic patients with haematological malignancies: a meta-analysis of randomised-controlled trials. Br J Haematol 2005;131(1):22–8.

188. Vazquez JA, Skiest DJ, Tissot-Dupont H, et al. Safety and efficacy of posaconazole in the long-term treatment of azole-refractory oropharyngeal and esophageal candidiasis in patients with HIV infection. HIV Clin Trials 2007;8(2):86–97.

189. Chakrabarti A, Chatterjee SS, Rao KL, et al. Recent experience with fungaemia: change in species distribution and azole resistance. Scand J Infect Dis 2009;41(4):275–84.

190. Maertens J, Marchetti O, Herbrecht R, et al. European guidelines for antifungal management in leukemia and hematopoietic stem cell transplant recipients: summary of the ECIL 3-2009 Update. Bone Marrow Transplant 2011;46(5):709–18.

191. Dodds-Ashley E. Management of drug and food interactions with azole antifungal agents in transplant recipients. Pharmacotherapy 2010;30(8): 842–54.

192. Lin JH. Drug-drug interaction mediated by inhibition and induction of P-glycoprotein. Adv Drug Deliv Rev 2003;55(1):53–81.

193. Moen MD, Lyseng-Williamson KA, Scott LJ. Liposomal amphotericin B: a review of its use as empirical therapy in febrile neutropenia and in the treatment of invasive fungal infections. Drugs 2009;69(3):361–92.

194. Noel GJ. Liposomal amphotericin B for empirical therapy in patients with persistent fever and neutropenia. J Pediatr 1999;135(3):399.

195. Lortholary O, Desnos-Ollivier M, Sitbon K, et al. Recent exposure to caspofungin or fluconazole influences the epidemiology of candidemia: a prospective multicenter study involving 2,441 patients. Antimicrob Agents Chemother 2011;55(2):532–8.

196. Walsh TJ, Teppler H, Donowitz GR, et al. Caspofungin versus liposomal amphotericin B for empirical antifungal therapy in patients with persistent fever and neutropenia. N Engl J Med 2004;351(14): 1391–402.

197. Chamilos G, Lewis RE, Kontoyiannis DP. Delaying amphotericin B-based frontline therapy significantly increases mortality among patients with hematologic malignancy who have zygomycosis. Clin Infect Dis 2008;47(4):503–9.

198. Spellberg B, Walsh TJ, Kontoyiannis DP, et al. Recent advances in the management of mucormycosis: from bench to bedside. Clin Infect Dis 2009; 48(12):1743–51.

199. Flynn TR, Shanti RM, Levi MH, et al. Severe odontogenic infections, part 1: prospective report. J Oral Maxillofac Surg 2006;64(7):1093–103.

200. Rega AJ, Aziz SR, Ziccardi VB. Microbiology and antibiotic sensitivities of head and neck space infections of odontogenic origin. J Oral Maxillofac Surg 2006;64(9):1377–80.

201. Levi ME, Eusterman VD. Oral infections and antibiotic therapy. Otolaryngol Clin North Am 2011;44(1): 57–78.

What are the Lessons We Can Glean from a Review of Recent Closed Malpractice Cases Involving Oral and Maxillofacial Infections?

Steven M. Holmes, DDS, Debra K. Udey, BA*

KEYWORDS

- Maxillofacial infections • Oral infections
- Oral and maxillofacial surgery • Malpractice

OMS National Insurance Company (OMSNIC) was founded in 1988 to provide liability insurance for oral and maxillofacial surgeons. OMSNIC insures oral and maxillofacial surgeons (OMS) who are either fellows or members of the American Association of Oral and Maxillofacial Surgeons. Currently, OMSNIC insures more than 4700 OMS, which represents 83% of the OMS available for OMSNIC to insure.

With more than 10,090 closed claims, OMSNIC has the most complete and in-depth claims data for all oral and maxillofacial malpractice claims. When we subtract the Department of Professional Regulation (DPR), Employment Practices Liability, and claims opened for deposition assistance, the actual number of plaintiff claims is 8155. Overall, 8% of OMSNIC's claims are taken to trial, 12% are settled, and 80% are dismissed with no indemnity payment. More than 94% of all of the cases taken to trial either end with defense verdicts or result in an indemnity payment less than the amount the plaintiff would have accepted to settle the case before trial.

The statistics for infection claims are interesting. They range from deaths to DPR investigations and deposition assistance. The actual number of closed plaintiff malpractice cases involving infections in the history of OMSNIC is 600 (7.4%). Ten of the 600 cases, less than 1 every other year, have been death cases. Seventy-eight cases or 13% of the 600 closed claims have ended with indemnity payments. The largest infection indemnity payments to date are $990,000, $350,000, and $250,000. The smallest indemnity paid is $500. Seventeen of the 78 infection indemnity payments have been $100,000 or more. Sixteen of the 78 indemnity payments have been less than $10,000. OMSNIC has taken six infection cases to trial. All were cases that OMSNIC wanted to settle, but the plaintiff would not settle for a reasonable indemnity payment. All six, as anticipated, have been plaintiff verdicts. The indemnity amounts ranged from $200,000 to $0 (plaintiff verdict, no damages).

The type of damages claimed range from death, amputation, brain abscess with permanent

Risk Management, OMS National Insurance Company, 6133 North River Road, Suite 650, Rosemont, IL 60018-5173, USA
* Corresponding author.
E-mail address: debra.udey@omsnic.com

Oral Maxillofacial Surg Clin N Am 23 (2011) 601–607
doi:10.1016/j.coms.2011.07.010
1042-3699/11/$ – see front matter © 2011 Elsevier Inc. All rights reserved.

disability, additional surgeries, and reconstructive surgery to loss of wages and pain and suffering.

CASE EXAMPLES
Case 1

A 43-year-old healthy man was seen for consultation regarding symptomatic tooth number 17. He returned a week later for an office procedure and had erupted teeth numbers 16 and 17 removed while under general anesthesia. When he returned for a 1-week postoperative visit, he complained of hearing a loud crack and pain in the number 17 site. He was seen by an associate for the postoperative visit and was rescheduled to be seen by the primary surgeon. That appointment was 4 days later and included a panoramic radiograph and examination. The patient's occlusion and the radiograph were noted to be normal. The patient was discharged from the practice.

The patient returned 1 month after the operation with complaints of pain and a bad taste in his mouth from the number 17 site. The examination showed granulation tissue and drainage from the number 17 site. The extraction area was irrigated and a small bone spicule was removed. The patient was placed on oral penicillin V potassium (penicillin VK), 250 mg 4 times a day for 7 days.

The patient's symptoms evidently improved and he was not seen again for 3 weeks when he returned with continued drainage. He was placed on clindamycin (Cleocin), 150 mg 4 times a day for 7 days.

Nine weeks after the procedure, the patient returned with continued drainage and pain. At 10 weeks after the procedure, the patient underwent an office general anesthetic and debridement. The specimen was sent for pathology. The pathology report stated that the specimen was consistent with "osteomyelitis of mandible." Our insured continued the low-dose oral clindamycin for an additional 4 weeks. No radiographs had been taken since 11 days after the procedure.

At 14 weeks after the procedure, the clindamycin was discontinued and the patient was again discharged from the practice. He returned 2 weeks later with continued drainage and pain. Our insured placed the patient on clindamycin 300 mg 4 times a day for 7 days. At 17 weeks after the procedure, the clindamycin was decreased to 150 mg and the progress note stated, "paresthesia remains." This notation was the first notation of paresthesia in the patient's progress notes.

At 4.5 months after the procedure, the patient returned with increased swelling and drainage. He was again placed on oral clindamycin, 300 mg 4 times a day, but he did not improve.

At 5 months after the procedure, the patient finally lost confidence in our insured and was seen by another OMS for a second opinion. He was immediately admitted to the hospital for a computed tomography (CT) scan and infectious disease consultation with the diagnosis of osteomyelitis of the left mandible. He was placed on appropriate intravenous (IV) antibiotics and taken to surgery where he had a resection of the left angle of the mandible, rigid fixation plate, extraction of number 18, inferior alveolar nerve neurorrhaphy with Vicryl conduit, and maxillomandibular fixation.

The patient recovered from the osteomyelitis and healed with a satisfactory occlusion. He did have permanent paresthesia of the left inferior alveolar nerve, limited mandibular range of motion, loss of tooth number 18, and minor weakness of the mandibular branch of the left facial nerve.

The patient retained an attorney who filed a malpractice lawsuit against OMSNIC's insured. Some of the allegations included

- Failure to diagnose a left mandibular angle fracture at 1 week after procedure
- Failure to obtain culture and sensitivity reports
- Failure to obtain radiographs during the prolonged postoperative course
- Failure to obtain an infectious disease consultation early in the postoperative period
- Failure to diagnose and appropriately treat osteomyelitis, even when supplied with a pathology report with the correct diagnosis
- Negligently treating the patient for 5 months.

The initial demand was for $1 million.

OMSNIC's Claims Committee reviewed the insured's records. The records were found to be poor. The chart lacked any documentation of the rationale for removal of the erupted tooth number 17. The operative note stated, "ext 16, surgical removal of 17." There was no description of the surgery. The postoperative notes were very brief and illegible at times. The care provided to the patient was determined to be not defensible.

The claim was settled for $250,000 because of the poor record keeping and less-than-appropriate care rendered to the patient. Little was spent for defense costs because the case was determined to be one to settle; and we, therefore, spent only what was needed to effect a favorable settlement.

This case had a complete lack of documentation regarding the decision-making steps in the patient's care. If every patient visit was charted with a subjective, objective, assessment, plan

(SOAP) note, this would not occur. State medical and dental practice acts require that the patients' concerns, results of the patient examination, diagnosis, treatment options, and the possible risks and benefits of treatment and no treatment be charted. Charts must be documented so that a similar practitioner can read a physician's or dentist's chart and be able to understand and describe the course of treatment.

Case 2

A 47-year-old healthy woman was referred to an OMSNIC insured for removal of erupted carious teeth numbers 1 and 32. The accompanying periapical radiographs showed decay also in tooth number 31. Using an intravenous general anesthetic, teeth numbers 1 and 32 were removed as a same-day consult and surgery. The OMS charged for surgical extractions, but the operative note only described forceps delivery of the teeth. The patient was discharged to return as needed and given erythromycin (E-Mycin), 250 mg 4 times a day for 5 days.

Two weeks later, the patient returned with a complaint of persistent pain in the area of the number 32 extraction site. Our insured noted a "possible infection" or "pulpitis of #31" as possible causes for the pain. Clindamycin (Cleocin), 300 mg 3 times a day for 10 days, was prescribed. The patient returned 2 days later with the same complaint of pain and now had soft tissue swelling. Under local anesthesia, the number 32 site was explored, irrigated with chlorhexidine gluconate 0.12% (Peridex), and a dry socket dressing placed. The clindamycin was increased to 4 times a day.

The patient returned 1 day later with diarrhea and no decrease in her pain complaint. A panoramic radiograph was obtained. Our insured saw no abnormalities on the film. The dry socket dressing was removed and the site was irrigated again. The clindamycin dosage was decreased to 150 mg 4 times a day and metronidazole (Flagyl), 500 mg 4 times a day for 10 days, was prescribed.

The patient returned a few days later, now 3 weeks after the procedure, without improvement. Under local anesthesia, the number 32 socket was curetted; the chart note read: "an abundance of inflamed tissue and multiple pieces lingual bone fragments, removed." No specimen was sent for pathology. Three days later, the patient was a little better, the clindamycin was discontinued, and the patient was referred to her dentist for the treatment of number 31.

The dentist referred the patient for endodontic treatment of number 31. The endodontist thought the prognosis for number 31 was guarded and

the patient chose extraction. Now more than 5 weeks since the removal of number 32, the patient returned to our insured OMS with the same symptoms. Number 31 was extracted using an intravenous anesthetic.

Four days later, at 6 weeks after the extraction of number 32, the patient returned with a complaint of pain in number 30. Our insured noted: "Sensitive to all lower right teeth, most likely due to inflammation of Inferior Alveolar Nerve." The patient was discharged from the practice and told to call if she did not continue to improve. There was no effort to investigate the continued pain and soft tissue swelling.

This patient was keeping a diary of her ongoing problems. After the office visit at 6 weeks after the procedure, she wrote in her electronic journal: "Bad pain in teeth. Dr X said it is nerve trauma and it would take time to heal itself. Says we can't do anything but wait and let it heal and settle down. He says that the bone was infected so that is also aggravating the nerve so until the bone infection goes away the nerve will still be upset. Call him if it doesn't seem get better." At OMSNIC's Claims Committee's review, it seemed that the patient had a better handle on the situation than did our insured.

Two weeks later, at 8 weeks after the procedure, the patient spent 9 hours in the hospital emergency department because of the pain in her right mandible. She had a CT scan done. The CT scan impression was "periostitis and mild destructive changes of the right hemimandible, consistent with osteomyelitis." The patient was seen again in our insured's office the following day. The OMS obtained a new panoramic radiograph and performed another debridement of the number 32 site while under local anesthesia, finding purulence and bone fragments. Again no specimen was sent for pathologic review. Flagyl, 500 mg 4 times a day for 10 days, was prescribed. The OMS did *not* obtain a copy of the CT report or go to the hospital to review the films.

At 9 weeks after the procedure, the patient had soft tissue swelling, purulence, and mobility of her right mandibular teeth around the midline to number 23. Our insured referred her to a periodontist with a new panoramic radiograph, which our insured likely did not review before the patient left the office. The periodontist extracted number 23 and began periodontal therapy.

When seen in the OMS office at 10 weeks after the procedure, the patient was noted to have induration and tenderness of the right floor of the mouth. She was started on Azithromycin (Z-pak) and Flagyl as oral antibiotics. The patient called the next day with a complaint of pain under her chin and was told to see her primary care physician for an ear, nose, and throat (ENT) referral. Our insured did not see the patient again. Her primary care physician referred her to an oral medicine/pain specialist who immediately diagnosed an active infection and referred her to an ENT physician.

She was admitted to the hospital and placed on IV antibiotics. After 3 days with no improvement, another OMS was consulted. The second OMS diagnosed acute osteomyelitis. Plain films and a panoramic radiograph demonstrated significant radiolucent changes extending from the number 32 extraction site to tooth number 20. An infectious disease physician was consulted. The second OMS took the patient to surgery to debride the mandible. The patient lost teeth numbers 20 through number 30. She completed an appropriate culture-guided IV antibiotic therapy course and recovered without additional surgery.

The patient retained an attorney and filed a medical negligence lawsuit against the OMSNIC insured OMS. The complaint included

- Negligently failed to properly and timely care for an infection which plaintiff developed
- …result of such negligence, the infection worsened and spread to the entire right body of the mandible
- Plaintiff required extensive surgery to address the infection
- …leaving plaintiff, age 47 years, with no teeth in her lower mouth except three on her left side. Plaintiff will require extensive reconstructive surgery.

The initial demand was $299,000.

The records of the insured, the subsequent treater, and the hospital were reviewed by OMSNIC's Claims Committee and independent expert reviewers. The insured's records were found to be somewhat illegible; but, once transcribed, they were thought to document the patient's experience in the OMS office. But it was obvious that the OMS did not consider the possibility of a significant infection or osteomyelitis. At the deposition, the OMS testified that he did not think that a patient who was not immunocompromised could develop osteomyelitis.

The case had some significant negative factors:

- Repeated explorations and debridements without cultures or specimens to pathology
- Did not obtain the CT report from the patient's emergency department visit
- Did not identify significant radiographic changes on at least 2 of his own follow-up panoramic radiographs.

This case finally settled at mediation for an indemnity payment of $60,000, with defense costs approaching $100,000.

Infection Cases Involving Death of the Patient

Two of the 10 death cases follow. They both involve the removal of third molars on young healthy patients. Some of the details of both patients' unfortunate deaths are unknown. The cases never became lawsuits because the OMS records supported the care rendered. Hospital records remained unavailable to OMSNIC.

Case 3

A 20-year-old healthy man was seen for consultation regarding removal of his third molars. He returned and the surgery was accomplished without complication.

Two days later, his family called the OMS office and reported that he was swollen and having difficulty swallowing. They were instructed to come to the office immediately. Examination noted bilateral swelling, maybe only a little more than usual. The OMS thought that the patient may have been developing a cellulitis, so the plan was to admit the patient to the hospital for IV antibiotics and hydration. While a hospital bed was assigned, the OMS began an IV line in the office and administered IV clindamycin (Cleocin) and hydrated the patient. The hospital bed was made available at 6 PM.

During the first 2 days in the hospital, the patient's condition remained stable. The nursing staff called the OMS at 7 PM the second night and told him the patient was having difficulty swallowing and breathing. The patient was transferred to the intensive care unit (ICU) where he was intubated. A CT scan was done and showed abscess formation and possibly necrotizing fasciitis. The OMS attempted to transfer the patient to a larger hospital, but the transfer was refused. The patient was taken to surgery for bilateral submandibular space abscess drainage. In the surgical suite, the patient had a cardiac arrest secondary to septic shock. He was successfully resuscitated. The patient was then transferred to the larger hospital.

Early the following morning, a diagnosis of abdominal compartment syndrome was made, and the patient died 3 hours later.

Case 4

A 17-year-old healthy girl from a rural town some distance from the OMS office was seen for a same-day consultation and removal of her impacted third molar teeth. The surgery was accomplished uneventfully with IV sedation.

On the second postoperative day, the family called with concern about swelling of the face and neck. The patient had no complaint of pain. They were told that this should be the height of the swelling and to call back if the swelling did not decrease.

The family called again on the fourth postoperative day to report that the swelling was not better. They were asked to come to the office. During the drive to the OMS office, the patient complained of dizziness. On arrival, she was placed into a wheelchair to enter the office. She then became unresponsive and looked bluish. An airway was placed and 100% oxygen was administered. The patient regained consciousness, the emergency medical services (EMS) system was activated, and monitors were placed. Her S_aO_2 was in the 80s. The EMS personnel attempted to start an IV, but were unsuccessful. She was transferred to the hospital.

She was diagnosed with group A streptococcus sepsis, dehydration, odontogenic infection; and she succumbed to acute renal failure.

LESSONS LEARNED FROM THE REVIEW OF CLOSED CLAIMS

When an OMS sees patients in his or her office who present with an infection for a second opinion, the usual course is to obtain studies and institute aggressive care. When an OMS sees patients in a hospital setting with a postoperative infection or preexisting odontogenic infection, the treatment is usually the same. However, patients who experience infections secondary to care rendered by the OMS in his or her office sometimes receive a different level of treatment.

The review of OMSNIC's infection claims data looking for recurrent trends shows that infection claims generally fall into 2 categories. The first involves the OMS who has a difficult time recognizing a significant postoperative infection in his or her own patients. The second involves patients who come into the office with a preexisting significant odontogenic infection. Although the diagnosis and planned treatment are appropriate for these patients, there are other issues that come into play that can derail the care and lead to a less-than-optimal outcome.

Surgeons recognize that dealing with patients who have postoperative problems is not one of the most rewarding ways to spend their time. Perhaps that is what sometimes leads to complacency. For example, a patient develops a nagging postoperative problem. The initial treatment performed was routine, the postoperative problem is not thought to be that serious, and the surgeon is reluctant to institute aggressive treatment. The prescribed antibiotic does not clear the infection, so the antibiotic is continued and the treatment turns into a prolonged course. Osteomyelitis is not on the radar, and the connection is not made that this could be the patient's diagnosis.

Unfortunately, what often happens in these situations is that patients finally lose confidence in their OMS and go to another practitioner, often their dentist. Seeing something amiss, the dentist refers the patients to another OMS. That surgeon jumps all over the problem with radiographic studies and a referral to an infectious disease specialist, and patients are appropriately treated. But the end result may be a claim for a failure to diagnose and properly treat the infection brought against the first OMS.

How can this scenario be avoided? One OMS office instituted an efficient course of action to deal with this type of situation. If after 3 postoperative visits the patient's problem was not resolved, the office scheduled the patient to be reevaluated by another OMS in the practice. The reevaluation included (1) a radiograph of the affected area; (2) a review of the chart, including the temperature trend of the patient (taken on all postoperative visits); (3) questioning the patient on his or her progress (whether there was improvement with antibiotic therapy or when dressings were changed and for how long); and (4) an assessment of whether the symptoms and treatment rendered supported the postoperative diagnosis or whether there could be another diagnosis.

A fresh assessment or independent evaluation of the patients' current status is imperative to prevent complacency. No matter what kind of evaluation process a surgeon has, it is important that a definitive process be in place so that patients do not languish in a prolonged postoperative course without a resolution of the problem. It is crucial to keep an open mind and to not let tunnel vision prevent the consideration of anything other than the working diagnosis. All too often antibiotics are prescribed for patients who have a seemingly nondescript and minor infection; and because the surgeon has decided it is a minor infection, the treatment instituted is not reviewed and no changes are made, even when patients continue to return. There is a reluctance to entertain any other diagnosis and patients languish. Meanwhile, the minor infection may really be an osteomyelitis that may progress to a fracture, loss of additional teeth, additional surgery, hospitalization, medical expenses, loss of wages, and pain and suffering. The progression sounds like the germination of a malpractice lawsuit.

When the surgeon conscientiously and aggressively follows patients with a postoperative infection and the infection clears or osteomyelitis is diagnosed and appropriately treated, patients usually appreciate the OMS's attentive care. There is much less likelihood of a claim as opposed to the situation where the OMS downplays the significance of the postoperative problem.

The second type of claim involves patients who present with a significant odontogenic infection. The problem in this type of case is not the diagnosis, which is usually fairly clear. These claims come from the cases where patients want to direct their care. Money is often the issue that almost always leads to the problem in the first case: lack of appropriate dental care. Patients were negligent in their own dental care, and then try to convince the OMS to take a less aggressive (less expensive) treatment plan. Patients may claim to not be able to afford radiographs or the CT scan and hospitalization for IV antibiotics, which will put the doctor in a difficult situation. There is always the desire to help patients and explore a less expensive way to render the needed treatment. The OMS may attempt to refer patients to the university hospital or the county trauma hospital, but patients may convince the OMS to undertake treatment as an office procedure or in the local hospital.

This benevolent attitude, although laudable, can lead to a disaster. The less than successfully treated infection may worsen and lead to more problems. Patients may talk the surgeon into treating them in the office or at the local hospital, when the appropriate course of action would be to refer them to a major hospital with a higher level of care. The anesthesia staff, OMS, and ICU staff in the local hospital may not be accustomed to seeing these very serious head and neck infections. Patients, who could not afford the treatment of a significant infection, are now faced with a more serious problem: inexperienced staff and more costs they cannot afford when their life is on the line. Then who is to blame?

Patients accepting personal responsibility is certainly on the decline in our patient population. Patients are not going to take responsibility for their choices. The finger will surely be pointed at the doctor who rendered substandard care. Will the OMS records even begin to support what ended up being inadequate care? Frequently, our insureds will admit wanting to refer patients but not doing so because of the patients' request. In the eyes of the plaintiff's attorney and the jury, the OMS is the learned doctor; patients could not make their own decisions in the face of a significant infection, therefore, the OMS made the decisions. The OMS will be judged by the decisions he or she made.

These types of situations can be very difficult. Surgeons cannot refuse to see patients in the hospital, and they do not want to render care that is less than the standard. It is paramount to treat patients in a manner that is consistent with the OMS's clinical judgment. It is also hoped that options can be worked out through the hospital to obtain the care needed for patients.

How patients are treated and what is said to patients is as important as the treatment rendered. Above all, jousting, which is defined as the criticism of another practitioner, should be avoided. Care must be taken when patients present with an odontogenic infection, whether referred before or after treatment. Sometimes the tendency is to assume that the previous care was not appropriately rendered, which accounts for the patients' condition, especially if the previous treating OMS is a competitor. The second OMS must remember that patients may go to a third OMS, and then he or she is in the same boat with the first OMS.

However, some patients are prescribed the appropriate treatment by their OMS but do not comply with it. This situation leads to the condition that the second opinion surgeon observes but was not the result of substandard care. Surgeons should be aware of this and not make any disparaging remarks about the care rendered before patients come to their office.

An untoward remark may imply or tell patients that they were the recipients of inadequate care. The OMS who makes the remark must remember that he or she is now treating those patients. If patients subsequently bring a claim for damages against the first OMS, the second OMS is likely to get dragged into it. Thus, the remark that set off the ultimate claim may come back to bite the one who uttered it.

One underlying component of treatment is the documentation of the care provided. This component cannot be ignored. When surgeons are treating patients with postoperative infections, cryptic notes, such as "patient no better" or "dressing changed," do not adequately describe the patients' clinical course. It is difficult, indeed, to defend the seeming lack of attention to the patients' situation with this type of note. Surgeons should write or dictate a complete progress note for each patient visit. The SOAP format is best, and even a short SOAP note can give a good picture of the situation. Good, legible, complete records in the SOAP format may dissuade the plaintiff's attorney from continuing the case. On the other hand, incomplete, cryptic, and illegible records encourage the continuation of the lawsuit because the plaintiff's attorney knows that even if the care rendered was appropriate, there is no documentation of those facts and the insurance company may be forced to settle a defensible claim.

In OMSNIC's experience, frequently the subsequent treating OMS has clear, legible, concise progress notes. The primary OMS is often his or her worst enemy. The records are all that the plaintiff's attorney or a jury has to evaluate the surgical and diagnostic skills of the OMS. In a trial, the jury is trying to decide if they would receive appropriate, compassionate care from the OMS if they were the patient.

In the courtroom, the plaintiff's attorneys will display the defendant's records against the records of the patient's subsequent treater or physician, which are detailed, legible, and in a SOAP format. The jury must choose between the injured patient's story and the OMS's records to try to determine if the OMS is a good surgeon. The records are incredibly important in the defense of a malpractice claim.

SUMMARY

OMS occasionally face significant infections in their own postoperative patients and with new patients who present with odontogenic infections to their offices or to hospital emergency departments. All of these patients need to be evaluated with a fresh approach to appropriately diagnose the infection and institute appropriate care at each visit because they are not routine patient appointments. This care may involve consultation with other physicians or another OMS.

The costs of care cannot overshadow the ultimate outcome for patients because care directed at decreasing patient costs rarely results in improved patient outcomes. The worst outcome for patients may be death, and for the OMS, an ugly, public, costly, and time-consuming malpractice case. Do for patients what you would want done for you or your family in similar circumstances.

The only defense the OMS has to possibly prevent or defend a malpractice claim in the face of an untoward outcome in an infection case is the quality of his or her records documenting the decision making that led to the patient's treatment or the lack of treatment. That is the major lesson OMSNIC has learned. This practice is what you would want a physician or dentist treating you or your family to do. Do not do less for patients.

The chart notes need to record patients' subjective concerns; the presenting signs and symptoms; the examination of patients at every visit; diagnosis; ordering and recording of diagnostic studies and results, including the radiographs taken in the office; and obtaining appropriate consultations, even if that means another OMS.

Recording the assessment of patients' conditions and the plan for treatment at every patient encounter would allow OMSNIC to defend the OMS treatment, when defensible. If OMS would embrace the golden rule, to treat all patients and record the chart entries in the same manner that they would want done for themselves or their family, they would not only provide appropriate care for their patients but have the documentation to prove it.

The 2 summarized death cases demonstrated appropriate patient care and record keeping. The cases involved the death of young healthy patients with their whole life ahead of them. Neither became a lawsuit. The parents of the patient in the second death case published an announcement in the town's newspaper that read in part: "To the oral surgeon that removed our daughter's wisdom teeth, we do not hold you responsible in any way. We know that you provided the most professional and gentle care possible and if our son needed any oral surgery, you would be the first person we would contact. We ask the community not to blame or judge any person in any way. God needed our angel to be his angel."[1] It is hoped that the lessons learned from these statistics and cases are taken to heart to help the OMS population see fewer infection claims.

REFERENCE

1. Bozeman Chronicle, Dec. 19, 2006.

Index

Note: Page numbers of article titles are in **boldface** type.

doi:10.1016/S1042-3699(11)00160-9

United States Postal Service

Statement of Ownership, Management, and Circulation
(All Periodicals Publications Except Requester Publications)

1. Publication Title	2. Publication Number	3. Filing Date
Oral and Maxillofacial Surgery Clinics of North America	0 0 6 - 3 6 2	9/16/11

4. Issue Frequency	5. Number of Issues Published Annually	6. Annual Subscription Price
Feb, May, Aug, Nov	4	$329.00

7. Complete Mailing Address of Known Office of Publication (Not printer) (Street, city, county, state, and ZIP+4®)

Elsevier Inc.
360 Park Avenue South
New York, NY 10010-1710

Contact Person
Amy S. Beacham
Telephone (Include area code)
215-239-3687

8. Complete Mailing Address of Headquarters or General Business Office of Publisher (Not printer)

Elsevier Inc., 360 Park Avenue South, New York, NY 10010-1710

9. Full Names and Complete Mailing Addresses of Publisher, Editor, and Managing Editor (Do not leave blank)

Publisher (Name and complete mailing address)

Kim Murphy, Elsevier, Inc., 1600 John F. Kennedy Blvd. Suite 1800, Philadelphia, PA 19103-2899

Editor (Name and complete mailing address)

John Vassallo, Elsevier, Inc., 1600 John F. Kennedy Blvd. Suite 1800, Philadelphia, PA 19103-2899

Managing Editor (Name and complete mailing address)

Barbara Cohen-Kligerman, Elsevier, Inc., 1600 John F. Kennedy Blvd. Suite 1800, Philadelphia, PA 19103-2899

10. Owner (Do not leave blank. If the publication is owned by a corporation, give the name and address of the corporation immediately followed by the names and addresses of all stockholders owning or holding 1 percent or more of the total amount of stock. If not owned by a corporation, give the names and addresses of the individual owners. If owned by a partnership or other unincorporated firm, give its name and address as well as those of each individual owner. If the publication is published by a nonprofit organization, give its name and address.)

Full Name	Complete Mailing Address
Wholly owned subsidiary of	4520 East-West Highway
Reed/Elsevier, US holdings	Bethesda, MD 20814

11. Known Bondholders, Mortgagees, and Other Security Holders Owning or Holding 1 Percent or More of Total Amount of Bonds, Mortgages, or Other Securities. If none, check box ☐ None

Full Name	Complete Mailing Address
N/A	

12. Tax Status (For completion by nonprofit organizations authorized to mail at nonprofit rates) (Check one)
The purpose, function, and nonprofit status of this organization and the exempt status for federal income tax purposes:
☐ Has Not Changed During Preceding 12 Months
☐ Has Changed During Preceding 12 Months (Publisher must submit explanation of change with this statement)

PS Form 3526, September 2007 (Page 1 of 3 (Instructions Page 3)) PSN 7530-01-000-9931 PRIVACY NOTICE: See our Privacy policy in www.usps.com

---

13. Publication Title		14. Issue Date for Circulation Data Below	
Oral and Maxillofacial Surgery Clinics of North America		August 2011	

15. Extent and Nature of Circulation		Average No. Copies Each Issue During Preceding 12 Months	No. Copies of Single Issue Published Nearest to Filing Date
a. Total Number of Copies (Net press run)		2255	1868
b. Paid Circulation (By Mail and Outside the Mail)	(1) Mailed Outside-County Paid Subscriptions Stated on PS Form 3541. (Include paid distribution above nominal rate, advertiser's proof copies, and exchange copies)	1458	1347
	(2) Mailed In-County Paid Subscriptions Stated on PS Form 3541 (Include paid distribution above nominal rate, advertiser's proof copies, and exchange copies)		
	(3) Paid Distribution Outside the Mails Including Sales Through Dealers and Carriers, Street Vendors, Counter Sales, and Other Paid Distribution Outside USPS®	210	215
	(4) Paid Distribution by Other Classes Mailed Through the USPS (e.g. First-Class Mail®)		
c. Total Paid Distribution (Sum of 15b (1), (2), (3), and (4))	▶	1668	1562
d. Free or Nominal Rate Distribution (By Mail and Outside the Mail)	(1) Free or Nominal Rate Outside-County Copies Included on PS Form 3541	69	58
	(2) Free or Nominal Rate In-County Copies Included on PS Form 3541		
	(3) Free or Nominal Rate Copies Mailed at Other Classes Through the USPS (e.g. First-Class Mail)		
	(4) Free or Nominal Rate Distribution Outside the Mail (Carriers or other means)	69	58
e. Total Free or Nominal Rate Distribution (Sum of 15d (1), (2), (3) and (4))	▶		
f. Total Distribution (Sum of 15c and 15e)	▶	1737	1620
g. Copies not Distributed (See instructions to publishers #4 (page #3))		518	248
h. Total (Sum of 15f and g)	▶	2255	1868
i. Percent Paid (15c divided by 15f times 100)		96.03%	96.42%

16. Publication of Statement of Ownership

☐ If the publication is a general publication, publication of this statement is required. Will be printed ☐ Publication not required
in the November 2011 issue of this publication.

17. Signature and Title of Editor, Publisher, Business Manager, or Owner

Amy S. Beacham - Senior Inventory Distribution Coordinator

Date September 16, 2011

I certify that all information furnished on this form is true and complete. I understand that anyone who furnishes false or misleading information on this form or who omits material or information requested on the form may be subject to criminal sanctions (including fines and imprisonment) and/or civil sanctions (including civil penalties).

PS Form 3526, September 2007 (Page 2 of 3)

Moving?

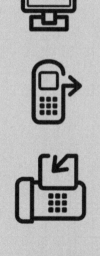

Printed and bound by CPI Group (UK) Ltd, Croydon, CR0 4YY

03/10/2024

01040346-0019